1998-1999

Pocket Book of Pediatric Antimicrobial Therapy

THIRTEENTH EDITION

1998-1999

Pocket Book of Pediatric Antimicrobial Therapy

THIRTEENTH EDITION

John D. Nelson, MD
Professor Emeritus of Pediatrics
The University of Texas
Southwestern Medical Center at Dallas
Southwestern Medical School
Dallas, Texas

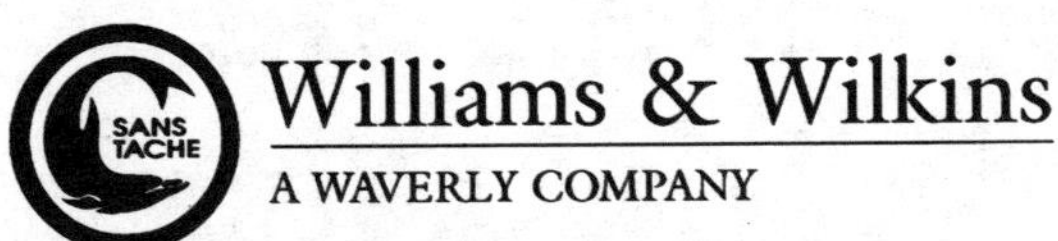

BALTIMORE • PHILADELPHIA • LONDON • PARIS • BANGKOK
BUENOS AIRES • HONG KONG • MUNICH • SYDNEY • TOKYO • WROCLAW

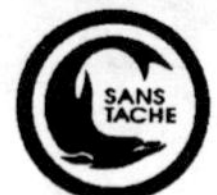

Editor: Jonathan W. Pine, Jr
Managing Editor: Leah Ann Kiehne Hayes
Marketing Manager: Peter Darcy
Production Coordinator: Raymond E. Reter
Project Editor: Lisa J. Franko
Printer & Binder: Vicks Lithograph & Printing, Yorkville, New York

351 West Camden Street
Baltimore, Maryland 21201-2436 USA

Rose Tree Corporate Center
1400 North Providence Road
Building II, Suite 5025
Media, Pennsylvania 19063-2042 USA

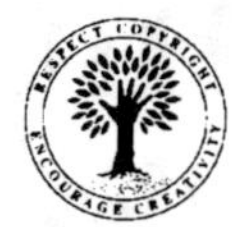

Accurate indications, adverse reactions, and dosage schedules for drugs are provided in this book, but it is possible that they may change. The reader is urged to review the package information data of the manufacturers of the medications mentioned.

Printed in the United States of America

First Edition, 1975

ISBN 0-683-30484-4

The publishers have made every effort to trace the copyright holders for borrowed material. If they have inadvertently overlooked any, they will be pleased to make the necessary arrangements at the first opportunity.

97 98 99 00 01
1 2 3 4 5 6 7 8 9 10

CONTENTS

I. INTRODUCTION TO THE THIRTEENTH EDITION

The field of infectious disease is a dynamic one with constant growth and change. New diseases are discovered, new antimicrobials are introduced, older antibiotics lose their utility for certain diseases but sometimes find new applications, and microbes find ways to escape the action of antimicrobials. Every two years when I revise this book, I wonder at the extent of changes that are necessary.

I appreciate greatly the helpful criticisms and suggestions of my infectious disease colleagues at The University of Texas Southwestern Medical Center: Doctors George McCracken, Trudy Murphy, Octavio Ramilo, Pablo Sánchez, Jane Siegel, and Loretta Wubbel. I extend special thanks to John Bennett for reviewing the antifungal section and to Pablo Sánchez for help with the newborn section. Tammy Bratton, PharmD provided information on drug dilutions.

Recent editions of this book have been translated into Chinese, German, Greek, Indonesian, Italian, Polish, Portuguese and Spanish. The task of the translators is complicated by the variability of drug availability in different countries. Fortunately, the major antimicrobials are universally available.

The large number of related drugs means that multiple options are available for a great many diseases. To avoid cluttering up and expanding the book I have indicated only one or two options for treating most infections. Clearly, other regimens might be suitable.

Some dosages and indications differ from those in the manufacturers' package inserts. In such situations the dosages recommended in this book have been found by controlled studies or by clinical experience to be efficacious and safe.

The continued popularity and apparent usefulness of this little book is gratifying. As in the past, I encourage readers to send suggestions for its improvement to me.

John D. Nelson, MD

II. CHOOSING AMONG AMINOGLYCOSIDES, BETA-LACTAMS, AND MACROLIDES

New drugs should be compared with others in the same class regarding (1) antimicrobial spectrum, (2) degree of potency within the spectrum, (3) pharmacokinetic properties, (4) demonstrated efficacy in clinical trials, (5) tolerance, toxicity and side effects, and (6) cost. If there is no substantial benefit in any of those areas, one should opt for using the older, more familiar drug because of the risk of unexpected adverse effects inherent in any new product.

Aminoglycosides. Five aminoglycosidic antibiotics are available in the U.S. as major drugs for coliform bacillary infections: amikacin, gentamicin, kanamycin, netilmicin, and tobramycin. (Streptomycin and spectinomycin have limited uses.) Resistance of Gram-negative bacilli to aminoglycosides is caused by adenylating, acetylating, or phosphorylating enzymes produced by the bacteria which inactivate the antibiotic. The specific activities are highly variable. As a result, antibiotic susceptibility tests must be done for each aminoglycoside drug separately. Kanamycin is not effective against *Pseudomonas aeruginosa* so the others are preferred whenever that infection is present or suspected. There are small differences in comparative toxicities of these aminoglycosides to the kidneys and eighth cranial nerve. In animal models netilmicin is the least toxic. It is possible that netilmicin and tobramycin are the safest, but there are conflicting reports in studies focusing on small changes in renal function rather than on frank renal failure. It is uncertain whether or not these small differences are clinically significant. In any case, it is advisable to monitor peak and trough serum concentrations in all patients; elevated peak and trough concentrations correlate with toxicity. Desired peak concentrations with amikacin and kanamycin are 20–35 μg/ml and trough concentrations less than 10 μg/ml; for the others they are 5–10 μg/ml and less than 2 μg/ml, respectively. Patients with cystic fibrosis require larger than normal dosage to achieve therapeutic serum concentrations, and they excrete aminoglycosides more rapidly. **Once Daily Dosing.** Once daily dosing of 5-6 mg/kg gentamicin or tobramycin have been used in some children; peak serum concentrations are greater than those achieved with thrice daily dosing. Regimens giving the daily dosage as a single infusion, rather than as traditional split doses every 8 hours, are safe and effective in adults and may be less toxic. Experience with once-daily dosing in children is limited to date, but it may become the standard after further experience. In the case of nosocomial infection, the choice among aminoglycosides should be based on knowledge of local susceptibility patterns. In addition to routine monitoring of *in vitro* susceptibility testing results to detect emergence of resistant strains, the policy of switching among the drugs for routine hospital use every one to two years might minimize the likelihood of resistance due to selective drug pressure.

Oral Cephalosporins (Cefaclor, cefadroxil, cefixime, cefpodoxime, cefprozil, ceftibuten, cefuroxime axetil, cephalexin, cephradine, and loracarbef). As a class, the oral cephalosporins have the advantages over oral penicillins of somewhat greater safety and greater palatability of the suspension formulations. (Penicillins have a bitter taste.) Cefuroxime and cefpodoxime, which are esters, are the least palatable. Cephalexin and cephradine have virtually identical properties and effectiveness, and they can be used interchangeably. The half-lives of cefadroxil, cefpodoxime, cefprozil, ceftibuten, and loracarbef in serum are about twice as long as those of the other drugs. This pharmacokinetic feature accounts for the fact that they can be given in only one or two daily doses. Cefaclor, cefixime, cefpodoxime, cefprozil, ceftibuten, loracarbef and cefuroxime have the advantage of adding *Haemophilus influenzae* (including beta-lactamase-producing strains) to the spectrum.

Parenteral Cephalosporins. First generation cephalosporins (cefazolin, cephalothin, cephapirin, cephradine) have been used mainly as back-up drugs for treatment of Gram-positive infections because their Gram-negative spectrum is limited. Cefazolin is tolerated best on intramuscular injection; furthermore, it is given q8h because of its longer half-life in serum rather than on the q4–6h schedules used for the others. Differences in the frequencies of vein irritation among the group are minor.

The second generation cephalosporins (cefamandole and cefuroxime) and a cephamycin (cefoxitin) added to the antibacterial spectrum. Cefoxitin has good activity against *Bacteroides fragilis* and can be used in place of chloramphenicol or clindamycin when that organism is implicated in disease. Cefotetan has a spectrum similar to that of cefoxitin but a longer serum half-life, so it can be given q12h. Cefamandole and cefuroxime added *Haemophilus influenzae* to the spectrum of cephalosporins. However, cefamandole is somewhat unstable to the TEM1 beta-lactamase elaborated by *H. influenzae*. This combined with its rather poor penetration into cerebrospinal fluid resulted in cases of *Haemophilus* meningitis developing in infants being treated with cefamandole. Cefuroxime is more stable to the enzyme and has better penetration into CSF (comparable to that of ampicillin). It has been used to treat meningitis due to the usual pathogens; however, reports of delayed sterilization of CSF limit its use for meningitis. Cefuroxime has utility as single drug therapy (in place of combinations such as nafcillin and chloramphenicol) for infants and young children with pneumonia, bone and joint infections or other conditions in which Gram-positive cocci and *Haemophilus* are the usual pathogens. Because of the substantial decrease of *Haemophilus influenzae* type b following adoption of routine immunization of infants against that organism, this advantage of cefuroxime is less important than in the past. Cefonicid has a prolonged serum half-life so that doses can be given every 12–24 hours. Cefonicid is not approved for use in children.

Among the many so-called "third generation" cephalosporins, cefoperazone and cefepime are not yet approved for use in children. All have enhanced potency against many Gram-negative bacilli, usually including aminoglycoside-resistant organisms. They are inactive against enterococci and *Listeria* and have variable activity against *Pseudomonas* and *Bacteroides*. Cefotaxime and ceftriaxone have been used successfully to treat meningitis caused by the usual pathogens. Limited experience with ceftazidime and ceftizoxime suggests that they too are effective for meningitis. These drugs have greatest usefulness for treating Gram-negative bacillary infections when aminoglycosides are contraindicated or when the organisms are resistant to customarily used drugs. Because cefoperazone and ceftriaxone are excreted to a large extent via the liver, they can be used with little dosage adjustment in patients with renal failure. Ceftazidime has the unique property of activity against

Pseudomonas aeruginosa that is comparable to that of the aminoglycosides. Ceftriaxone has a serum half-life of 4–7 hours and can be given once or twice a day.

Penicillinase-resistant Penicillins (Cloxacillin, dicloxacillin, methicillin, nafcillin, oxacillin). Nafcillin differs pharmacologically from the others in being excreted primarily by the liver rather than by the kidneys. This may be the reason for its lack of nephrotoxicity. Nephrotoxicity or hemorrhagic cystitis occurs in 5% of children treated with methicillin. For this reason nafcillin is preferred over methicillin for parenteral use with two exceptions: neonates and patients with hepatic disease. Nafcillin pharmacokinetics in the newborn are erratic, especially in jaundiced babies; furthermore, methicillin nephrotoxicity is rare in the neonate. Nafcillin pharmacokinetics are also erratic in persons with liver disease. For oral use, cloxacillin, oxacillin and dicloxacillin are essentially equivalent, but the latter has the greatest anti-staphylococcal activity in vitro.

Anti-pseudomonal Penicillins and Carbapenems (Imipenem, meropenem, mezlocillin, piperacillin, ticarcillin, ticarcillin-clavulanate). Piperacillin is the most active in vitro against *Pseudomonas*. Mezlocillin does not affect platelet adhesiveness significantly, but the others do; this could be an advantage in patients who have another risk factor for bleeding. In general, *Pseudomonas* strains resistant to ticarcillin are resistant to the newer drugs. These drugs should be used along with an aminoglycoside or cephalosporin for treating *Pseudomonas* infections in compromised hosts for synergistic effect. Timentin® is the combination of ticarcillin and the beta-lactamase inhibitor, clavulanate, and Zosyn® is the combination of piperacillin with tazobactam, another beta-lactamase inhibitor. The combinations have little effect on activity against *Pseudomonas* but do extend the spectrum to many beta-lactamase-positive bacteria. Imipenem and meropenem are carbapenems with a broader spectrum of activity than any other beta-lactams currently available. Imipenem is not approved by the FDA for use in children but meropenem is. At present they are recommended for treatment of infections caused by bacteria resistant to most other drugs. Imipenem has CNS toxicity, especially in patients with meningitis, but this has not been a problem to date with meropenem.

Aminopenicillins (Amoxicillin, amoxicillin-clavulanate, ampicillin, ampicillin-sulbactam, bacampicillin). Bacampicillin is rapidly and completely converted in the body to ampicillin so it is an indirect means of administering ampicillin. Bacampicillin is the most efficiently absorbed so peak blood concentrations are greater than after the same dosage of amoxicillin or ampicillin. Ampicillin is more likely than the others to cause diarrhea and to disturb colonic coliform flora and cause overgrowth of *Candida*. Augmentin® is a combination of amoxicillin and clavulanate for oral use that permits amoxicillin to be active against many beta-lactamase-producing bacteria. Sulbactam, another beta-lactamase inhibitor, is combined with ampicillin in the parenteral formulation, Unasyn®. Clinical experience is too limited to date to assess its role in pediatric patients.

Monobactams. The only monobactam licensed for use in the U.S. is aztreonam. Its spectrum is similar to that of the anti-*Pseudomonas* aminoglycosides so the clinical indications are similar. Experience with the drug is insufficient to know for which clinical situations, if any, that it might replace the aminoglycosides.

Macrolides. Erythromycin is the prototype of a class called macrolide antibiotics. Almost thirty macrolides have been produced, but only four are commercially available in the U.S.: erythromycin, azithromycin, clarithromycin and dirithromycin. (Azithromycin is actually an azalide compound structurally similar to macrolides.) As a class these drugs achieve greater concentrations in tissues than in serum. (Tissue concentrations are markedly greater with azithromycin and clarithromycin than with erythromycin.) As a result, measuring serum concentrations is clinically not useful. Erythromycin has poor gastrointestinal tolerance in many patients. This is less of a problem with the newer drugs. Erythromycin suspensions are ester formulations and must be hydrolyzed to the active base compound. The estolate form results in greater serum and tissue concentrations of erythromycin than do the other esters. Macrolides have the broadest range of antimicrobial activity of all classes of antibiotics. This is especially true of azithromycin and clarithromycin, which are demonstrating clinical utility in *Haemophilus influenzae,* chlamydial, and mycobacterial infections that is greater than that of erythromycin.

III. ANTIBIOTIC THERAPY FOR NEWBORNS

A. RECOMMENDED THERAPY FOR SELECTED CONDITIONS

NOTE: To avoid repetition, the recommended dosages and intervals of administration of antibiotics indicated with an asterisk in most of the following conditions are given in the Table on pages 16 and 17.

Condition	Therapy	Comment
Congenital syphilis	Aqueous penicillin G 50,000 u/kg q 12h (day of life 1–7), q8h (> 7 days) IV OR procaine penicillin G G 50,000 u/kg IM once daily; x 10–14 days; Optional alternative for asymptomatic infant or when infants' nontreponemal test is negative: benzathine penicillin G 50,000 u/kg IM, single dose	Obtain follow-up serology at 3, 6, 12 mos until nontreponemal test nonreactive or decreased 4-fold
Congenital toxoplasmosis	Sulfadiazine 100 mg/kg/day PO div q6-12h AND pyrimethamine 2 mg/kg PO daily x 2 (loading dose), then 1 mg/kg PO once daily for 6 weeks; Alternative: pyrimethamine (as above) AND clindamycin*	Supplemental folinic acid 5–10 mg 3 times weekly; Therapy for 6-12 months may be indicated
Herpes simplex infection	Acyclovir 30 mg/kg/day as 1–2 hr IV infusion div q8h OR vidarabine 15–30 mg/kg/day as 12 hour or longer IV infusion x 10 days; PLUS trifluridine ophthalmic sol'n topically q2h for conjunctivitis (max 9 times/day)	Larger dosages of acyclovir (45–60 mg/kg/day) and 14-21 days of Rx may be used for disseminated or CNS disease
Human immunodeficiency virus infection	Zidovudine 8 mg/kg/day PO div q6h OR 6 mg/kg/day IV div q6h; x 6 weeks (Consult with HIV specialist)	For infants born to HIV-positive mothers
Tetanus neonatorum	Penicillin G* IV x 10 days	Antitoxin and sedation; Do not use IM injections

Parotitis, suppurative	Oxacillin* IV AND aminoglycoside IV, IM x 10 days	Usually staphylococcal but occasionally coliform
Conjunctivitis		
- Chlamydial	Erythromycin* estolate or ethylsuccinate PO x 10–14 days OR topical erythromycin, tetracycline or sulfacetamide ointment q.i.d.	Erythro PO preferable to topical therapy because NP carrier state eradicated; Treat mother and her sexual partner
- Gonococcal	Ceftriaxone 50 mg/kg/day (max 125 mg) IV, IM once daily OR cefotaxime 50 mg/kg/day IV, IM div q12h; x 7 days (A single dose of ceftriaxone may be effective in uncomplicated infection)	Chloramphenicol or tetracycline ophthalmic drops or ointment optional; Treat mother and her sexual partner; Evaluate for chlamydial infection
- *Staphylococcus aureus*	Oxacillin* IM, IV x 7–10 days	Additionally: Neomycin ophthalmic drops or ointment
- *Pseudomonas aeruginosa*	Ticarcillin* or mezlocillin* IV, IM AND aminoglycoside* IM, IV x 7–10 days (Alternative: ceftazidime*)	Polymyxin B ophthalmic drops or ointment; Subtenon or subconjunctival antibiotics in some cases
Gastrointestinal infections		
- *Salmonella*	Cefotaxime* IV, IM x 7–10 days if suspected sepsis or focal infection	Observe for focal complications (meningitis, arthritis, etc.)

* See pages 14–15 for dosage

Condition	Therapy	Comment
Gastrointestinal infections (cont'd.)		
- Necrotizing enterocolitis or peritonitis secondary to bowel rupture	Ticarcillin* IV, IM AND aminoglycoside* IM, IV x 10 days or longer; cefotaxime* suitable alternative to aminoglycoside; Vancomycin* IV if *Staphylococcus epidermidis* or methicillin-resistant staphylococcus cultured; common alternative: vancomycin* + aminoglycoside* ± clindamycin*	Bacteremia in 30–50% of cases; After 2–3 days of age *Bacteroides* common in gut; Clindamycin* or metronidazole* for ticarcillin-resistant *Bacteroides fragilis*
Sepsis and meningitis	NOTE: Duration of therapy: 7–10 days for sepsis without a focus; 21 days minimum for Gram-negative meningitis	
- Initial therapy, organism unknown	Ampicillin* IV AND aminoglycoside* IV, IM	Ampicillin* AND cefotaxime* is a suitable alternative, especially if aminoglycoside-resistant nosocomial organism suspected
- *Bacteroides fragilis* spp. *fragilis*	Metronidazole*, clindamycin*, mezlocillin* or ticarcillin* IV, IM	Metronidazole preferred for CNS infection
- Coliform bacteria	Cefotaxime* IV, IM; Lumbar intrathecal or intraventricular injections of aminoglycoside are not beneficial in usual case	Aminoglycoside* is suitable alternative
- Group A	Penicillin G* IV	
- Group B streptococcus	Ampicillin* or penicillin G* IV AND gentamicin* IV IM (Discontinue gentamicin when strain known to be fully susceptible to ampicillin and sterilization achieved)	Synergy may be advantage especially against penicillin-tolerant strains

- Enterococcal sp.	Vancomycin* IV <u>AND</u> aminoglycoside* IV, IM	
- Gonococcal	Ceftriaxone 50 mg/kg/day IV, IM once daily <u>OR</u> cefotaxime 100 mg/kg/day IV, IM div q12h	Penicillin G* for susceptible strains
- *Listeria monocytogenes*	Ampicillin* IV, IM <u>AND</u> aminoglycoside* IV, IM	Aminoglycosides synergistic *in vitro* with ampicillin
- *Staphylococcus epidermidis*	Vancomycin* IV	Usually methicillin-resistant
- *Staphylococcus aureus*	Oxacillin* IV, IM; Vancomycin* IV for methicillin-resistant *Staphylococcus*	Vancomycin preferred for meningitis
- *Pseudomonas aeruginosa*	Mezlocillin* or ticarcillin* IV, IM <u>AND</u> aminoglycoside* IV, IM	Ceftazidime* is a suitable alternative
Osteomyelitis, suppurative arthritis		Surgical drainage of pus; Physical therapy
- Gonococcal arthritis and tenosynovitis	Ceftriaxone* IV, IM x 7–10 days (penicillin G* IV if organism susceptible)	
- *Staphylococcus aureus*	Oxacillin* IV, IM x 21 days minimum; Vancomycin* IV for methicillin-resistant *Staphylococcus*	Change to penicillin G if organism susceptible
- Coliform bacteria	Cefotaxime* <u>OR</u> aminoglycoside* IV, IM x 21 days minimum	Cephalosporins better than aminoglycosides for deep tissue infection

* See pages 14-15 for dosage

NEWBORN

NEWBORN

Condition	Therapy	Comment
- Group B streptococcus	(See Group B streptococcal meningitis)	
- Unknown	Oxacillin* IV, IM AND cefotaxime* IV, IM x 21 days minimum	
Otitis media	Few controlled treatment trials in newborns; Suggest using initial therapy as for older infants (See page 22); If no response, obtain middle ear fluid for culture	Cephalosporin or Augmentin may have advantage because of activity vs. coliforms and Staph (10–20% of cases)
- Coliform bacteria	Cefaclor 30–40 mg/kg/day PO div q8–12h x 10 days OR Augmentin (same dosage)	Aminoglycoside* or cefotaxime* if parenteral therapy needed
- *Staphylococcus aureus*	Cloxacillin or cephalexin 50 mg/kg/day PO div q6–8h x 10 days	Oxacillin* if unable to treat PO
- Streptococcus	Penicillin V 30 mg/kg/day PO div q8h x 10 days	May be given IV
- *Haemophilus*	Cefaclor 30–40 mg/kg/day PO div q8–12h OR amoxicillin 30–40 mg/kg/day PO div q8–12h if susceptible	Other regimens not tested in neonates
Pulmonary infections		
- *Staphylococcus aureus*	Oxacillin* IV, IM x 21 days minimum; Vancomycin* IV for methicillin-resistant Staph	Closed tube drainage of empyema
- *Pseudomonas aeruginosa*	Mezlocillin* or ticarcillin* IV, IM AND aminoglycoside* IV, IM x 14 days or longer	Ceftazidime* is a suitable alternative
- Group B streptococcus	Penicillin G* IV OR ampicillin* IV, IM x 10–14 days	Radiograph often mimics hyaline membrane disease
- *Chlamydia trachomatis*	Erythromycin* PO x 14–21 days	Ampicillin, amoxicillin or sulfa drugs may be effective

- Aspiration pneumonia	Oxacillin* IV, IM <u>AND</u> aminoglycoside* IV, IM x 7–10 days	Most aspiration episodes are not followed by pneumonia and do not require antibiotic therapy
- Pertussis	Erythromycin* x 5–10 days <u>OR</u> ampicillin* IV, IM if PO meds not retained	Usually acquired from parent or other adult in household
Skin and soft tissues		
- Impetigo neonatorum	Cleansing alone <u>OR</u> oxacillin* IV, IM <u>OR</u> cephalexin 50 mg/kg/day PO div q6–8h <u>OR</u> mupirocin topically; x 5 days	No antibiotic for superficial impetigo; Chlorhexidine baths; Break lesions with alcohol swab
- Erysipelas (and other Group A streptococcal infections)	Penicillin G* IV x 5–7 days	Group B streptococcus may produce similar cellulitis or nodular lesions
- Breast abscess	Oxacillin* IV, IM x 5–7 days; aminoglycoside* <u>OR</u> cefotaxime* if Gram-negative rods seen in pus	Gram stain of expressed pus/colostrum or I&D material; (Avoid damage to breast tissue)
- *Staphylococcus*	Oxacillin* IV, IM x 5–7 days; Vancomycin* for methicillin-resistant *Staphylococcus*	Value of systemic antibiotics over surgical drainage alone not established
- Group B streptococcus	Penicillin G* IV <u>OR</u> ampicillin* IV, IM; x 5–7 days	Usually no pus formed
- Coliform bacteria	Aminoglycoside* or cefotaxime* IM, IV x 5–7 days	

* See pages 14–15 for dosage

Condition	Therapy	Comment
Skin and soft tissues (cont'd.) - Omphalitis and funisitis		
Group A or B streptococci	Penicillin G* IV x 5–7 days OR (for Group A strep) benzathine penicillin G 50,000 u/kg IM x 1 dose PLUS topical "triple dye" or bacitracin ointment	Group A strep usually causes "wet cord" without pus and with minimal erythema
Staphylococcus aureus	Oxacillin* IV, IM x 5 days or longer	Observe for bacteremia and other focus of infection
Necrotizing funisitis	Oxacillin* IV, IM AND aminoglycoside* IV, IM	Unknown etiology but secondary infection may occur
Clostridial	Penicillin G* IV x 10 days or longer	Crepitance and rapidly spreading cellulitis around umbilicus
Urinary tract infection	Initial empiric therapy usually with ampicillin* and gentamicin* pending culture and susceptibility test results	Investigate for abnormalities of urinary tract
- Coliform bacteria	Gentamicin* IV, IM OR amikacin* IV, IM x 10 days	Ampicillin used for *Proteus mirabilis* infection
- *Pseudomonas aeruginosa*	Mezlocillin* or ticarcillin* IV, IM AND aminoglycoside* IV, IM x 10 days	Ceftazidime* is a suitable alternative
- Enterococcus	Ampicillin* IV, IM AND aminoglycoside* x 10 days	Vancomycin if ampicillin-resistant

* See pages 14-15 for dosage

B. USE OF ANTIMICROBIALS DURING PREGNANCY OR BREASTFEEDING

A number of factors determine the degree of transfer of antibiotics across the placenta: lipid solubility, degree of ionizatio molecular weight, protein binding, placental maturation, and placental and fetal blood flow. During the latter part of pregnanc maternal serum concentrations of most antibiotics decrease because of the increased volume of distribution. Fetal serur concentrations of the following drugs are equal to, or only slightly less than, those in the mother: penicillin G, amoxicillin, ampicilli carbenicillin, methicillin, sulfonamides, trimethoprim, tetracyclines, nitrofurantoin, and chloramphenicol. The aminoglycosid concentrations in fetal serum are from 20–50% of those in maternal serum. Cephalosporins, nafcillin, oxacillin, clindamycin, an colistimethate penetrate poorly (10–15%) and fetal concentrations of erythromycin and dicloxacillin are less than 10% of those i the mother.

Some drugs can cause harm to the pregnant woman or fetus. Drugs that are contraindicated are: ribavirin, amantadin cinoxacin, ciprofloxacin, norfloxacin, erythromycin estolate, griseofulvin, nalidixic acid, tetracyclines, emetine, lindane, an primaquine. Drugs that are considered safe are: penicillins, aztreonam, cephalosporins, erythromycin base, methenami mandelate, spectinomycin, nystatin, chloroquine, niclosamide, paromomycin, permethrin, praziquantel, pyrantel pamoate, an pyrethrins. Drugs not listed should be used with caution for firm clinical indications (The Medical Letter 1987;29:61).

Concentrations of antibiotics in human breast milk are not well studied. Isoniazid, metronidazole, trimethoprim an sulfonamides occur in equal concentrations in maternal serum and milk. Tetracyclines, chloramphenicol, and erythromycin ar found in breast milk in concentrations 50–75% of those in serum. Breast milk concentrations of penicillin G and V aminoglycosides, nalidixic acid, oxacillin, novobiocin, various cephalosporins, and nitrofurantoin have been reported to be less tha 25% of the maternal serum concentrations. Because these are microgram amounts, they would not be ingested by the infant i therapeutic amounts.

For example, if an infant took 110 cc/kg body weight of breast milk containing 10 mcg/ml isoniazid in a day, this woul amount to a "dose" of 1.1 mg/kg/day. The same infant ingesting milk containing 10 mg/dl of sulfonamide would receive 1 mg/kg/day. On the other hand, with a penicillin V concentration of 0.1 mcg/ml in breast milk, the amount of penicillin taken in b the infant would be only 0.011 mg/kg/day.

The AAP Committee on Drugs recommends that breast feeding may be discontinued 12–24 hours before treating a nursin mother with metronidazole. Other antibiotics are usually compatible with breast feeding, but it warns about the possibility o inducing hemolysis in babies with G-6-PD deficiency by nalidixic acid, nitrofurantoin or sulfa drugs. (Transfer of Drugs and Othe Chemicals into Human Milk. Pediatrics 1994;93:137)

NEWBORN

C. TABLE OF ANTIBIOTIC DOSAGES FOR NEONATES

Antibiotics	Routes of Administration	Dosages (mg/kg/day) and Intervals of Administration				
		Body Weight < 2000 g		Body Weight > 2000 g		
		0–7 days old	8-28 days old	0–7 days old	8-28 days old	> 28 days old
Ampicillin	IV, IM	100 div q 12h	150 div q 8h	150 div q 8h	200 div q 6h	200 div q 6h
Aztreonam	IV	60 div q 12h	90 div q 8h	90 div q 8h	120 div q 6h	120 div q 6h
Cefazolin	IV, IM	40 div q 12h	40 div q 12h	40 div q 12h	60 div q 8h	60 div q 8h
Cefotaxime	IV, IM	100 div q 12h	150 div q 8h	100 div q 12h	150 div q 8h	150 div q 6h
Ceftazidime	IV, IM	100 div q 12h	150 div q 8h	100 div q 8h	150 div q 8h	150 div q 8h
Ceftriaxone	IV, IM	50 once daily	50 once daily	50 once daily	75 once daily	100 once daily
Clindamycin	IV, IM, PO	10 div q 12h	15 div q 8h	15 div q 8h	20 div q 6h	30 div q 6h
Erythromycin	IV, PO	20 div q 12h	30 div q 8h	20 div q 12h	40 div q 8h	40 div q 6h
Metronidazole	IV, PO	15 div q 24h	15 div q 12h	15 div q 12h	30 div q 12h	30 div q 6h
Mezlocillin	IV, IM	150 div q 12h	225 div q 8h	150 div q 12h	225 div q 8h	300 div q 6h
Nafcillin	IV	50 div q 12h	75 div q 8h	75 div q 8h	150 div q 6h	150 div q 6h
Oxacillin	IV, IM	100 div q 12h	150 div q 8h	150 div q 8h	200 div q 6h	200 div q 6h
Penicillin G	IV	100,000 U div q 12h	225,000 U div q 8h	150,000 U div q 8h	200,000 U div q 6h	200,000 U div q 4h
Procaine Penicillin G	IM	50,000 U q 24h	50,000 U q 24h	50,000 U q 24h	50,000 U q 24h	50,000 U q 24h

DRUGS FOR NEONATES DOSED ACCORDING ONLY TO AGE

Drug	Routes of Administration	Dosage (mg/kg/DOSE) Gestational Age Plus Weeks of Life			
		≤ 26 Wks	27-34 Wks	35-42 Wks	≥43 Wks
Acyclovir	IV	10 q 12h	10 q 12h	10 q 8h	10 q 8h
Amikacin[a]	IV, IM	7.5 q 24h	7.5 q 18h	10 q 12h	10 q 8h
Gentamicin[b]	IV, IM	2.5 q 24h	2.5 q 18h	2.5 q 12h	2.5 q 8h
Tobramycin[b]	IV, IM	2.5 q 24h	2.5 q 18h	2.5 q 12h	2.5 q 8h
Vancomycin[c]	IV	15 q 24h	15 q 18h*	15 q 12h*	15 q 8h*

[a]Desired serum concentrations: 20-30 mcg/ml (peak), < 10 mcg/ml (trough)
[b]Desired serum concentrations: 5-10 μg/ml (peak), < 2.5 μg/ml (trough)
[c]Desired serum concentrations: 20-40 μg/ml (peak), < 10 μg/ml (trough)

*At 28 days of life (4 wks) vancomycin is dosed at 20 mg/kg/dose. The interval remains the same.

(Table prepared by Pablo J. Sánchez, MD)

IV. ANTIMICROBIAL THERAPY ACCORDING TO CLINICAL SYNDROMES

NOTES:

1. This tabulation should be considered a rough guideline for the "usual" patient. Deviations should be made according to physiologic peculiarities of the patient. Dosages recommended are for patients with normal or nearly normal hydration, renal function and hepatic function. See Section XII for information on patients with impaired renal function and Section XV for dosages based on square meters of body surface area.
2. Duration of treatment should be individualized. The periods recommended are based on common practice and general experience. Critical evaluations of duration of therapy have been carried out in very few diseases.
3. Diseases are arranged by body systems. Consult the index for the alphabetized listing of diseases and Section VII for the alphabetized listing of etiologic agents and for uncommon agents not included in this section.

Clinical Diagnosis	Therapy	Comments
A. SKIN AND SOFT TISSUE INFECTIONS		NOTE: Erythromycin for penicillin-allergic patients
Streptococcal cellulitis (erysipelas)	Penicillin G 50,000–100,000 u/kg/day, IV div q4–6h initially; then penicillin V 50 mg (80,000 u)/kg/day PO div q6–8h x 10 days	These dosages may be unnecessarily large but little clinical experience with smaller dosages
Lymphangitis, lymphadenitis, blistering dactylitis (streptococcal)	Penicillin V 25–50 mg (40,000–80,000 u)/kg/day PO div q6–8h OR erythromycin 40–50 mg/kg/day PO div q8–12h; x 10 days	For severe disease, penicillin IV (as above)
Impetigo	Mupirocin topically to lesions t.i.d.; OR (for extensive lesions) erythromycin (as above) or cefadroxil 30 mg/kg/day PO div q12h	Bathe daily; Usually mixed streptococcal and staphylococcal infection
Bullous impetigo, staphylococcal scarlet fever	Cefadroxil 30 mg/kg/day PO div q12h OR cloxacillin 50 mg/kg/day PO div q6h x 5–7 days	Other anti-staphylococcal drugs can be used

Scalded skin syndrome	Nafcillin or oxacillin 150 mg/kg/day IV div q6h initially; then cloxacillin OR cefadroxil (as above); x 5–7 days	Burow's or Zephiran compresses for intertriginous areas
Pyoderma, abscesses, cervical adenitis, Ludwig's angina (streptococcal, staphylococcal)	Cefadroxil OR cloxacillin (as above); x 5–10 days	I & D when indicated; Nafcillin IV for serious infections
Necrotizing fasciitis (streptococcal, staphylococcal)	Nafcillin or oxacillin 150 mg/kg/day IV div q6h x 10 days (Add aminoglycoside or ceftazidime if Gram-negative infection suspected)	Debridement; Watch for hypocalcemia, hypoproteinemia; Occasionally due to Gram-negative organisms
Buccal cellulitis (*Haemophilus*) **or cellulitis of unknown etiology**	Cefotaxime 100–150 mg/kg/day IV div q6h OR ceftriaxone 50 mg/kg IM, IV once daily; OR chloramphenicol 50–75 mg/kg/day IV div q6h; x 5–7 days	R/O meningitis; *Larger dosages needed for meningitis*
Suppurative myositis (Staphylococcal) (Syn: tropical myositis, pyomyositis)	Nafcillin or oxacillin 150 mg/kg/day IV div q6h x 7–10 days; Alternatives: other anti-staphylococcal beta-lactams, vancomycin	Surgical drainage or excision when needed
Gas gangrene (clostridial)	Penicillin G 250,000 u/kg/day IV div q4h x 10 days; Consider hyperbaric oxygen therapy	Antitoxin was of doubtful efficacy and is no longer available
Nontuberculous (atypical) mycobacterial adenitis	Total surgical excision is usually curative and antimicrobial therapy is not necessary in non-immunocompromised patient.	If surgical excision not possible, rifampin or clarithromycin therapy possibly effective
Tuberculous adenitis	As for pulmonary tuberculosis (See page 24)	Surgical excision usually not indicated

Clinical Diagnosis	Therapy	Comments
Animal and human bites	Augmentin 20–40 mg/kg/day PO div q8h x 5–7 days; For hospitalized patients use Timentin or ampicillin and clindamycin	Human bites often mixed aerobes and anaerobes; Consider rabies prophylaxis for animal bites; Tetanus prophylaxis
B. SKELETAL INFECTIONS		SEE SECTION XI FOR DISCUSSION OF ORAL ANTIBIOTIC THERAPY
Suppurative arthritis		Needle aspiration or surgical drainage; Physiotherapy
- Newborns	See Section III	
- Infants (*Haemophilus*, streptococci, *Staphylococcus*)	Cefuroxime or cefotaxime 100–150 mg/kg/day IV, IM div q8h OR (for streptococcus) pencillin G 100,000 u/kg/day IV div q4–6h x 14 days or longer OR (for *Staphylococcus*) nafcillin or oxacillin 150 mg/kg/day IV div q6h x 21 days or longer	*Haemophilus* unlikely in immunized populations
- Children (*Staphylococcus*, streptococci)	Nafcillin or oxacillin 150 mg/kg/day IV div q6h x 3 weeks or longer; Alternatives: other beta-lactams, clindamycin; vancomycin for methicillin-resistant staphylococci	Change to penicillin G if streptococcus or susceptible pneumococcus
- Gonococcal arthritis or tenosynovitis	Ceftriaxone 50 mg/kg once daily IV, IM OR (if susceptible) penicillin G 100,000 u/kg/day IV div q6h x 7–10 days	3–5 days therapy adequate in adults, but not tested in children
- Other bacteria	See Section V for preferred antibiotics	

Osteomyelitis or osteochondritis		Surgery; Immobilization
- Newborn	See Section III	
- Acute, initial therapy (usually *Staphylococcus*, streptococci, *Haemophilus*)	Infants: cefuroxime or cefotaxime 100–150 mg/kg/day IV, IM div q8h; Children > 4 yrs: nafcillin or oxacillin 150 mg/kg/day IV, div q6h x 3 weeks or longer. Alternatives: other beta-lactams, clindamycin	In children add ceftazidime to nafcillin if Gram-negative rods in pus, pending culture and susceptibility results
- Acute, other organisms	See Section V for preferred antibiotics	
- *Pseudomonas aeruginosa*	Ceftazidime 150 mg/kg/day IV, IM div q8h OR mezlocillin or ticarcillin 200–300 mg/kg/day IV div q6h AND (compromised host) gentamicin 6–7.5 mg/kg/day IM, IV or amikacin 15–20 mg/kg/day IM, IV div q8h; x 10 days	If thorough surgical debridement not done, longer therapy required
- Chronic (staphylococcal)	Dicloxacillin 75–100 mg/kg/day PO div q6h OR cephradine/cephalexin 100–150 mg/kg/day PO div q6h; x 6–12 months	Surgery; Monitor serum for bactericidal titer or antibiotic concentration (See Section X[illegible] for details)

C. EYE INFECTIONS

Hordeolum (sty) or chalazion	None (Topical antibiotic not necessary)	Warm compresses; I & D when necessary
Acute conjunctivitis	Polymyxin B-bacitracin or sulfacetamide ophthalmic drops q2h or ointment q4–6h	See page 7 for chlamydial, gonococcal, pseudomonal infection
Herpetic conjunctivitis	Trifluoridine sol'n 1 drop q2–3h while awake x 7–14 days; OR vidarabine ointment topically q3h until 1 week after healing	Consider steroids if keratitis present (Refer to ophthalmologist)

Clinical Diagnosis	Therapy	Comments
Periorbital cellulitis (Pre-septal infection)		
- Associated with sinusitis	Cefuroxime or cefotaxime 100–150 mg/kg/day IV, IM div q 8h x 5–7 days	Follow with oral antibiotic (See page 23)
- Idiopathic (*Haemophilus* or pneumococcal)	Cefuroxime or cefotaxime 100–150 mg/kg/day IV, IM div q8h OR chloramphenicol 50–75 mg/kg/day IV div q6h; x 7–10 days; Vancomycin for penicillin-resistant pneumococcus	Lumbar puncture to R/O meningitis; LARGER DOSAGES NEEDED FOR MENINGITIS
- Associated with periorbital skin lesion (streptococcal, staphylococcal)	Nafcillin or oxacillin 150 mg/kg/day IV div q6h x 7–10 days	Oral anti-staphylococcal antibiotic for less severe infection
Orbital cellulitis (Post-septal infection)	Nafcillin or oxacillin 150 mg/kg/day IV div q6h AND chloramphenicol 75–100 mg/kg/day IV div q6h x 10–14 days	Usually staphylococcal or Gram-negative bacilli; Surgical drainage of pus
Dacryocystitis	No antibiotic usually; when needed, based on Gram stain and culture of pus	Warm compresses; May require surgical probing of nasolacrimal duct
Endophthalmitis	NOTE: Subconjunctival/sub-tenon antibiotic often needed; steroids commonly used	
- Staphylococcal	Nafcillin or oxacillin 150 mg/kg/day IV div q6h x 10–14 days; Alternatives: other beta-lactams or vancomycin	Penicillin for susceptible organisms
- Pneumococcal, meningococcal	Penicillin G 250,000 u/kg/day IV div q4h x 10–14 days (vancomycin for penicillin-resistant pneumococci)	R/O meningitis

- Gonococcal	Ceftriaxone 50 mg/kg once daily IV, IM x 7 days or longer	
- *Pseudomonas*	Mezlocillin or ticarcillin 200–300 mg/kg/day IV div q4–6h AND gentamicin 6–7.5 mg/kg/day IM, IV or amikacin 15–20 mg/kg/day IM, IV div q8h x 10–14 days	Piperacillin or ceftazidime are alternatives
Retinitis		
- Cytomegalovirus	Ganciclovir OR foscarnet (See Section VIII for dosage)	
D. EAR AND SINUS INFECTIONS		
External otitis, bacterial	Optimal therapy unknown; cleaning canal of detritus important; antibiotic or antibiotic-steroid drops (e.g., Cortisporin suspension) customarily used but efficacy not proved	Wick moistened with Burow's sol'n used for marked swelling of canal; For "swimmer's ear," VoSol or alcohol-vinegar mixture to canal after water exposure
External otitis, fungal (otomycosis)	Topical 1/2 alcohol-1/2 vinegar sol'n OR 25% M-cresyl acetate (Cresylate) t.i.d.	Usually *Aspergillus*; Debride canal
Furuncle of external canal	Cefadroxil 30 mg/kg/day PO div q12h OR cloxacillin 50 mg/kg/day PO div q6–8h OR cephradine/cephalexin 50 mg/kg/day PO div q6–8h	I & D; Antibiotic not necessary unless cellulitis
Bullous myringitis	Antibiotics, as for otitis media with effusion (See the following entry)	Current concept is that this is simply one manifestation of acute otitis media
Otitis media, acute		
- Newborns	See Section III	

Clinical Diagnosis	Therapy	Comments
Otitis media, acute (cont'd) - Infants and children (pneumococcus, *Haemophilus*, *Moraxella* most common)	Amoxicillin or Augmentin 40 mg/kg/day PO div q8h <u>OR</u> erythromycin-sulfa combination 50 mg/kg/day of erythro component PO div q6–8h <u>OR</u> cefaclor 40 mg/kg/day PO div q8–12h <u>OR</u> TMP/SMX 8 mg/kg/day of TMP component PO div q12h <u>OR</u> cefixime 8 mg/kg once daily or div q12h <u>OR</u> cefprozil, cefuroxime axetil or loracarbef 30 mg/kg/day div q12h <u>OR</u> cefpodoxime 10 mg/kg/day div q12h <u>OR</u> ceftibuten 9 mg/kg once daily <u>OR</u> clarithromycin 15 mg/kg/day div q12h; x 5–10 days <u>OR</u> azithromycin 10 mg/kg (loading dose day 1) followed by 5 mg/kg q24h x 4 days	Gram stain and culture of pus if spontaneous rupture; If prior antibiotic therapy or compromised host, suspect unusual infection and do tympanocentesis for culture; Effective oral therapy for beta-lactam resistant pneumococci not established, but clindamycin or increased dosage of beta-lactams may be useful

<u>A Note on Acute Otitis Media with Effusion</u>: Several antibiotic regimens are effective for AOM. Customarily, amoxicillin is used initially and other drugs are given for amoxicillin failures or relapses. The physician should consider advantages and disadvantages regarding antibacterial spectrum, palatability of suspensions, and cost. TMP/SMX is not effective for Group A streptococcal infection. When prophylaxis is indicated, use amoxicillin or sulfa drug in one-half the therapeutic dose once or twice daily. How penicillin resistance in pneumococci affects empiric therapy is an unresolved issue.

Clinical Diagnosis	Therapy	Comments
Mastoiditis, acute (pneumococcus, staphylococcus, Group A streptococcus; *Haemophilus* rare)	Nafcillin or oxacillin 150 mg/kg/day IV div q6h OR cefuroxime 100–150 mg/kg/day IV, IM div q8h x 10 days; Alternatives: other beta-lactams or vancomycin for penicillin-resistant pneumococci	R/O meningitis; Surgery as needed; Change to oral therapy after clinical improvement
Mastoiditis, chronic	Antibiotics only for acute superinfections (according to culture of drainage); also, when chronic *Pseudomonas* infection, mezlocillin or ticarcillin 200–300 mg/kg/day IV div q4–6h x 5–7 days	Daily cleansing of ear important; After resolution, use amoxicillin or sulfa prophylaxis for otitis; If no response, surgery

Sinusitis, acute (*Haemophilus*, pneumococcus, streptococcus, *Moraxella*)	Same as for acute otitis media but 14–21 days may be needed	Sinus irrigations when indicated
E. NOSE AND THROAT INFECTIONS		
Diphtheria	Erythromycin 40–50 mg/kg/day PO div q6h x 14 days OR penicillin G 150,000 u/kg/day IV div q6h; PLUS antitoxin	Antitoxin available only from CDC (tel: 404-639-2889); Isolation until 3 daily nose and throat cultures negative
Streptococcal tonsillopharyngitis, scarlet fever and peritonsillar cellulitis	Penicillin V 25–50 mg/kg/day PO div q6–8h x 10 days OR benzathine penicillin 25,000 u/kg IM (max 1.2 million u) as a single dose; Alternatives: oral cephalosporins	Erythromycin or clindamycin for penicillin-allergic patients (Caution: ~5% of Group A strep resistant)
Epiglottitis (aryepiglottitis, supraglottitis) **or bacterial tracheitis**	Cefuroxime 100–150 mg/kg/day IV, IM div q8h OR chloramphenicol 50–75 mg/kg/day IV div q6h x 5–7 days; Alternatives: cefotaxime, ceftriaxone	Provide airway
Gingivostomatitis, herpetic	Acyclovir 15 mg/kg PO 5 times daily x 7 days (Give IV for severe disease)	Regimen reported effective in one study
Retropharyngeal or lateral pharyngeal cellulitis or abscess	Clindamycin 30 mg/kg/day PO, IV, IM div q6h OR nafcillin or oxacillin 150 mg/kg/day IV div q6h and chloramphenicol 50–75 mg/kg/day IV, PO	Usually aerobes and anaerobes; I & D when pus present; Consider tonsillectomy for peritonsillar abscess

Clinical Diagnosis	Therapy	Comments
F. LOWER RESPIRATORY INFECTIONS		
Respiratory syncytial virus infection (bronchiolitis, pneumonia)	Ribavirin 6 g vial (20 mg/ml in sterile water) aerosolized by SPAG-2 over 18–20 hr period daily x 3–5 days	Treat only for severe disease or patients with underlying cardiopulmonary disease
Pertussis	Erythromycin (estolate may be preferable) 50 mg/kg/day PO div q6h x 7 days (Re-administer vomited doses, or change to ampicillin 100 mg/kg/day IV, IM div q6h)	Hospitalize young babies; Avoid mist therapy; Avoid cough suppressants; Isolate until two daily cultures negative or for 10 days
Tuberculosis		
- Primary pulmonary	Isoniazid 10-15 mg/kg/day (max 300 mg) PO, IM x 6-9 mos AND rifampin 10–20 mg/kg/day (max 600 mg) PO, IV x 6-9 mos AND pyrazinamide 20-40 mg/kg/day PO x 2 mos; If in area with known drug resistance, add ethambutol 20 mg/kg/day PO OR streptomycin 30 mg/kg/day IM initially	Test for HIV infection; Directly observed therapy (DOT) preferred; After 1 month of therapy, can change to 2 x weekly dosing (Double dosage of INH and PYR; rifampin remains same dosage)
- Skin test conversion	Isoniazid 10–15 mg/kg/day (max 300 mg) PO daily x 6 months (12 months for immune compromised patients)	Single drug Rx if no clinical or radiographic evidence of disease
- Exposed infant < 4 yrs, or immunocompromised patient	Isoniazid 10–15 mg/kg PO daily x 3 mos after last exposure	If PPD remains negative and child well, stop prophylaxis
Lung abscess		
- Primary, putrid (i.e., foul-smelling)	Clindamycin 30 mg/kg/day PO, IM, IV div q6–8h; OR penicillin G 100,000 u/kg/day IV div q4–6h and chloramphenicol 50–75 mg/kg/day IV div q6h; x 10 days or longer	Usually polymicrobial infection with aerobes and anaerobes

- Primary, non-putrid	Cefuroxime 100–150 mg/kg/day IV, IM div q8h or other beta-lactamase-resistant beta-lactam; x 10 days or longer	Bronchoscopy necessary if abscess fails to drain; Surgical excision rarely necessary
- Secondary to other focus of infection (osteomyelitis, etc.)	Nafcillin or oxacillin 150 mg/kg/day IV div q6h x 10 days or longer OR other beta-lactams	Usually staphylococcal; cephalosporin for coliforms
Pneumonia in immunosuppressed, neutropenic host	Nafcillin or oxacillin 150 mg/kg/day IV div q6h or vancomycin 40 mg/kg/day IV div q6h (if methicillin-resistant Staph suspected) AND ceftazidime 150 mg/kg/day IV div q8h; Alternative: mezlocillin or ticarcillin 200–300 mg/kg/day IV div q6h AND amikacin 15–22.5 mg/kg/day or gentamicin 6–7.5 mg/kg/day IM, IV div q8h AND nafcillin (as above)	Consider opportunistic bacteria, pneumocystis, cytomegalovirus, fungi, tuberculosis; Biopsy or bronchoalveolar lavage of lung may be needed to establish diagnosis
Acute pulmonary exacerbations of cystic fibrosis	Ticarcillin 300–400 mg/kg/day IV div q4h AND tobramycin 6–10 mg/kg/day IM, IV div q6–8h; Alternatives: other anti-*Pseudomonas* beta-lactams and aminoglycosides OR ceftazidime 150 mg/kg/day IV div q8h OR ciprofloxacin 30 mg/kg/day PO, IV div q 8h; x 7–10 days	Larger than normal dosages of aminoglycosides required in most patients with cystic fibrosis; Monitor peak serum concentrations of aminoglycosides
***Pneumocystis carinii* pneumonia**	(See page 56)	
Bronchitis, acute	No antibiotic for most cases (viral); if bacterial infection suspected, use same drugs as for acute otitis or sinusitis (See page 22)	*Haemophilus, Moraxella*, pneumococcus most common pathogens in adults and (?) in children

Clinical Diagnosis	Therapy	Comments
Allergic bronchopulmonary aspergillosis	Prednisone 0.5 mg/kg every other day	Larger dosages may lead to tissue invasion
Pneumonia with empyema		Initial therapy based on Gram stain of empyema fluid
- Pneumococcal, Group A streptococcal	Penicillin G 150,000 u/kg/day IV div q4–6h x 10 days (Change to PO penicillin V in same dosage after clinical improvement); Alternatives: cephalosporins, clindamycin	Closed chest tube drainage of purulent fluid; Typically clinical improvement is slow
- Staphylococcal	Nafcillin or oxacillin 150 mg/kg/day IV div q6h OR vancomycin 40 mg/kg/day div q6h; x 21 days or longer (Alternatives: cephalosporins)	Closed chest tube drainage of empyema
- *Haemophilus influenzae* b or pneumonia of unestablished etiology (< 5 yrs of age)	Cefuroxime or cefotaxime 100–150 mg/kg/day IV, IM div q8h; OR ampicillin 150 mg/kg/day IV, IM div q6h and chloramphenicol 50–75 mg/kg/day IV div q6h OR ceftriaxone 50 mg/kg IV, IM once daily; x 10–14 days	Closed chest tube drainage; R/O meningitis; *Larger dosages needed for meningitis*
Lobar or segmental consolidation		
- *Haemophilus* or unknown etiology	Cefuroxime 100–150 mg/kg/day IV, IM div q8h x 10 days	Change to PO after improvement
- Pneumococcal	Penicillin G 150,000 u/kg/day IV div q4–6h x 10 days	Change to PO penicillin V in same dosage after improvement

- *Klebsiella pneumoniae*	Gentamicin 6–7.5 mg/kg/day IM, IV div q8h x 10 days or longer OR amikacin 15–20 mg/kg/day IM, IV div q8h (Alternative: cefotaxime 150 mg/kg/day IV, IM div q8h)	Suspect if distended lobe; Abscesses common but empyema rare
Bronchopneumonia		
- Mild to moderate illness	No antibiotic therapy unless epidemiological/clinical reasons to suspect specific pathogen other than virus	Most viral; Broad spectrum antibiotics increase risk of superinfection
- Serious, life-threatening illness	Initially, until etiology established, nafcillin or oxacillin 150 mg/kg/day IV div q6h AND gentamicin 6–7.5 mg/kg/day or amikacin 15–22.5 mg/kg/day IM, IV div q8h (cefotaxime or cefuroxime may be effective)	Needle aspiration of lung, tracheal aspirate or bronch-alveolar lavage for Gram stain and culture when indicated
Afebrile pneumonia syndrome of early infancy	Supportive, or (if chlamydia suspected) erythromycin 40 mg/kg/day PO div q6h x 14 days	Most viral or chlamydial; Often interstitial infiltrate
Other pneumonias of established etiology		
- *Chlamydia pneumoniae* (TWAR), *C. psittaci* or *C. trachomatis*	A macrolide OR tetracycline (pts > 7 yrs) (ampicillin for *C. trachomatis*)	For dosage, see Section VIII
- Cytomegalovirus	Ganciclovir (plus IV immune globulin)	For dosage, see Section VIII
- *E. coli, Enterobacter* spp.	An aminoglycoside or cephalosporin	For dosage, see Section VIII
- *Francisella tularensis*	Gentamicin or streptomycin	See page 40
- Fungi	Amphotericin B or combined therapy	For dosage, see Section VI

Clinical Diagnosis	Therapy	Comments
- Influenza A	Amantadine	For dosage, see page 38
- Legionnaires' disease	A macrolide and rifampin	For dosage, see Section VIII
- Melioidosis	See page 39	
- *Mycoplasma pneumoniae*	A macrolide or tetracycline	For dosage, see Section VIII
- *Paragonimus westermani*	Praziquantel	For dosage, see page 61
- *Pseudomonas aeruginosa*	Anti-*Pseudomonas* penicillin AND amino-glycoside OR ceftazidime	For dosage, see Section VIII
G. HEART INFECTIONS		
Purulent pericarditis		SURGICAL DRAINAGE OF PUS
- *Staphylococcus aureus*	Nafcillin or oxacillin 150 mg/kg/day IV div q6h OR (for methicillin-resistant staphylococci) vancomycin 40 mg/kg/day IV div q6h x 3 weeks or longer	Change to penicillin G if susceptible
- *Haemophilus influenzae* b	Cefuroxime 100–150 mg/kg/day IV, IM div q8h x 10–14 days; Alternatives: cefotaxime, ceftriaxone	Ampicillin for beta-lactamase-negative strains
- Pneumococcus, meningococcus, Group A streptococcus	Penicillin G 150,000 u/kg/day IV, IM div q4–6h x 10–14 days	(?) vancomycin for penicillin-resistant pneumococci
- Coliform bacilli	Cefotaxime 100–150 mg/kg/day IV, IM div q6–8h x 3 wks or longer; Alternatives: other cephalosporins, aminoglycoside	Alternative drugs depending on susceptibilities

- Tuberculous	(See page 24)	Corticosteroids for first 2–3 months
Endocarditis		
- Viridans streptococcus	Penicillin G 150,000 u/kg/day IV div q4–6h x 30 days (optional: AND streptomycin 30 mg/kg/day IM div q12h during first 14 days); OR vancomycin 40 mg/kg/day IV div q6h	Monitor serum bactericidal activity; See Section XI for discussion of oral therapy
- Enterococcus	Ampicillin 150 mg/kg/day IV, IM div q6h x 30 days AND gentamicin 6–7.5 mg/kg/day IM, IV div q8h; OR penicillin G 250,000 u/kg/day IV div q4–6h AND streptomycin 30 mg/kg/day IM div q12h; x 30 days	Longest experience with the penicillin-streptomycin regimen; Combined Rx used for synergistic bactericidal activity
- *Staphylococcus aureus*, *Staphylococcus epidermidis*	Nafcillin or oxacillin 150 mg/kg/day IV div q6h x 6 wks OR, for methicillin-resistant staphylococci, vancomycin 40 mg/kg/day IV div q6h; Consider adding rifampin or aminoglycoside for synergistic effect	Surgery may be necessary in acute phase; Avoid cephalosporins because of conflicting data on efficacy
- Pneumococcus, gonococcus, Group A streptococcus	Penicillin G 150,000 u/kg/day IV div q4–6h x 30 days (vancomycin for penicillin-resistant pneumococci)	Ceftriaxone for gonococcus until susceptibilities known
- Prophylaxis for:		**If penicillin allergy:**
- Dental, esophageal and upper respiratory procedures	Amoxicillin PO 50 mg/kg 1 hr before procedure OR Ampicillin IM, IV 50 mg/kg 30 min before procedure	Azithromycin or clarithromycin PO 15 mg/kg 1 hr before Clindamycin 20 mg/kg 30 min before (IV) or 60 min before (PO)

- Genitourinary and gastrointestinal procedures	Ampicillin IM, IV 50 mg/kg AND gentamicin IM, IV 1.5 mg/kg 30 min before; 6 hr later ampicillin IM, IV 25 mg/kg	Vancomycin IV 20 mg/kg over 1-2 hr AND gentamicin IM, IV
H. GASTROINTESTINAL INFECTIONS	(See Section VII for parasitic infections)	
***Helicobacter pylori* gastritis, peptic ulcer disease**	Clarithromycin 500 mg PO tid AND omperazole 40 mg PO once daily x 2 wks, followed by omperazole alone x 2 wks	Most data from studies in adults; other regimens include bismuth, amoxicillin, metronidazole
Shigellosis	Cefixime 8 mg/kg/day PO div 12-24 h x 5 days OR (for Pts > 18 yrs) ciprofloxacin 500 mg PO q12h	Trimethoprim-sulfamethoxazole, tetracycline, chloramphenicol, ampicillin, nalidixic acid when *Shigella* susceptible; Avoid anti-peristaltic drugs
Salmonellosis	Usually none for self-limited diarrhea OR amoxicillin 50 mg/kg/day PO div q8h x 5–7 days OR TMP/SMX as for shigellosis (See page 40 for typhoid fever)	Treat infants with bacteremia, compromised hosts and those with septic clinical picture or colitis (IV antibiotics for bacteremia)
Escherichia coli		
- Enteropathogenic	Neomycin 100 mg/kg/day PO div q6–8h	Most traditional "entero-pathogenic" strains not toxigenic or invasive
- Enterotoxigenic	Trimethoprim-sulfamethoxazole (as for shigellosis) OR neomycin or colistin PO	Most illnesses brief and self-limited
- Enteroinvasive	(?) Orally absorbable antibiotic, such as ampicillin, amoxicillin or trimethoprim-sulfamethoxazole	No controlled clinical trials on which to base a recommendation

Clinical Diagnosis	Therapy	Comments
"Turista" (traveler's diarrhea)	As for enterotoxigenic *E. coli* in the previous entry	50–75% of cases due to toxigenic *E. coli*; If not improved after 5 days, investigate for *Shigella*, *Giardia*, etc.
Yersinia enterocolitica	Antimicrobial therapy probably not of value	May mimic appendicitis
Campylobacter jejuni	Erythromycin 40 mg/kg/day PO div q6h x 5 days; Alternative (for adults): ciprofloxacin	Abdominal pain may mimic acute surgical abdomen
***Aeromonas* sp.**	(?) Trimethoprim-sulfamethoxazole as for shigellosis	Efficacy not established
Antibiotic-associated colitis	Metronidazole 30 mg/kg/day PO div q6h; Alternative: vancomycin 40 mg/kg/day PO div q6h x 7 days	Due to overgrowth of *Cl. difficile* in gut; Vancomycin may cause emergence of resistant enterococci in gut
Perirectal abscess	Clindamycin 30–40 mg/kg/day IV, PO div q6–8h AND aminoglycoside or cephalosporin	*S. aureus* common but may be mixed with coliforms, anaerobes; Surgical drainage
I. GENITOURINARY AND SEXUALLY TRANSMITTED INFECTIONS		*Consider testing for HIV infection in children with sexually transmitted diseases*
Genital herpes infection	Acyclovir 400 mg PO 3 x daily x 5 days (recurrent episode) OR acyclovir 200 mg PO 5 x daily x 7–10 days (first episode) OR (for severe disease) acyclovir 15 mg/kg/day as 1 hr IV infusion div q8h x 5–7 days	Most effective when started early in course of infection; For prevention of recurrence 400 mg 2 x daily

Clinical Diagnosis	Therapy	Comments
Urinary tract infection		
- Acute cystitis	Amoxicillin 30 mg/kg/day PO div q8h OR cefixime 8 mg/kg/day PO div q12-24h; x 7–10 days	*In vivo* susceptibility test: follow-up culture after 36–48 hrs treatment. If culture positive, change treatment according to *in vitro* susceptibilities
- Acute pyelonephritis	Gentamicin 6 mg/kg/day IV, IM div q8h OR trimethoprim-sulfamethoxazole 8 mg TMP–40 mg SMX/kg/day PO, IV div q12h; x 10 days	Parenteral drug if sepsis suspected; Change to appropriate oral drug after clinical response
- Prophylaxis for recurrent bacteriuria	Trimethoprim-sulfamethoxazole 2 mg TMP–10 mg SMX/kg PO q1–2 days OR nitrofurantoin 1–2 mg/kg PO q1–2 days at bedtime	Prophylaxis for patients with reflux or frequent infections
Epididymitis	Cefuroxime 100–150 mg/kg/day div q8h OR nafcillin 150 mg/kg/day IV div q6h and chloramphenicol 50–75 mg/kg/day IV, PO div q6h; x 7–10 days	Usually due to *Haemophilus* or *S. aureus* in young children; Treat as for gonorrhea and chlamydia in older children
Trichomoniasis	See Section VII	
Vaginitis or cervicitis		
- Vulvovaginal candidiasis	See Section VI	
- *Shigella*	As for diarrhea (See page 30)	50% have bloody discharge; Usually not associated with diarrhea

- Chlamydial	Doxycycline (patients > 7 yrs) 4 mg/kg/day (max 200 mg) PO div q12h x 7 days OR azithromycin 1 g PO as single dose	Alternatives: erythromycin, sulfisoxazole, amoxicillin
- Bacterial vaginosis (formerly "nonspecific vaginitis")	Metronidazole 500 mg PO twice daily x 7 days or as single 2 g PO dose; Alternative: intra-vaginal clindamycin cream or metronidazole gel	Caused by synergy of *Gardnerella* with anaerobes
Gonorrhea		
- Newborns	See Section III	
- Genital infections	Ceftriaxone 125 mg IM OR cefixime 400 mg PO OR azithromycin 2g PO (each as a single dose); Treatment regimens of demonstrated efficacy for children: 1) Procaine penicillin G 100,000 u/kg IM (max 4.8 mu) as single dose (two injection sites) AND probenecid 25 mg/kg PO (max 1 g) 2) Amoxicillin 50 mg/kg PO as single dose AND probenecid 25 mg/kg PO 3) Spectinomycin 40 mg/kg IM as single dose	Ceftriaxone preferred; Serologic test for syphilis; Repeat in 3 mos. if treated with something other than penicillin; Social evaluation re possibility of child abuse; Follow with treatment for presumed chlamydia
- Disseminated gonococcal infection	Ceftriaxone 50 mg/kg/day IM, IV once daily x 7 days	No controlled studies in children; Increase dosage for meningitis
Syphilis		See most recent CDC *Sexually Transmitted Diseases Treatment Guidelines*
- Congenital	See Section III	

- Primary, secondary	Benzathine penicillin G 2,400,000 u IM (approximately 50,000 u/kg) in 2 injection sites, single dose OR doxycycline 4 mg/kg/day (max 200 mg) PO div q12h x 14 days (Pts > 7 yrs)	Follow-up serologic tests at 3, 6 and 12 months; Do not use benzathine-procaine penicillin mixtures; Evaluate for possible sexual abuse
- Syphilis of more than 1 year duration	Benzathine penicillin G 2,400,000 u IM (50,000 u/kg) in 2 injection sites weekly for 3 doses	Optimal treatment schedule not established
Chancroid	Ceftriaxone 250 mg IM as single dose OR erythromycin 2 g/day PO div q6h x 7 days OR azithromycin 1 g PO as single dose	Serologic test for syphilis
Lymphogranuloma venereum (*Chlamydia trachomatis*)	Doxycycline 4 mg/kg/day (max 200 mg) PO (patients > 7 yrs) div q12h OR erythromycin 2 g/day PO div q6h; x 21 days	
Pelvic inflammatory disease	Cefoxitin 2 g IV q6h and doxycycline 100 mg PO bid OR clindamycin 900 mg IV q8h and gentamicin 1.5 mg/kg IV, IM q8h; (Other regimens include oxacillin, ciprofloxaxin, metronidazole)	Two drugs given until clinical improvement and followed by doxycycline alone to complete 14 days

J. CENTRAL NERVOUS SYSTEM INFECTIONS NOTE: IN AREAS WHERE PENICILLIN-RESISTANT PNEUMOCOCCI EXIST, INITIAL EMPIRIC THERAPY SHOULD BE WITH VANCOMYCIN PLUS CEFOTAXIME OR CEFTRIAXONE UNTIL SUSCEPTIBILITY TEST RESULTS AR AVAILABLE

Bacterial meningitis

NOTE: Dexamethasone (0.6 mg/kg/day IV div q6h x 4 days) as an adjunct to antibiotic therapy decreases hearing deficits and possibly other neurologic sequelae in *Haemophilus* meningitis and possibly other types. The first dose of dexamethasone is preferably given before the first dose of antibiotic.

Clinical Diagnosis	Therapy	Comments
- Neonatal	See Section III	
- *Haemophilus influenzae* b	Cefotaxime 200-300 mg/kg/day IV div q6h OR ceftriaxone either 100 mg/kg/day IV div q12h or 80 mg/kg IV, IM once daily; Alternative: ampicillin 200–400 mg/kg/day IV div q6h OR chloramphenicol 100 mg/kg/day IV div q6h; x 10 days	Chloramphenicol can be given PO; Rifampin prophylaxis for patients and contacts (for susceptible strains) according to Red Book recommendations
- Pneumococcus	For penicillin-resistant pneumococci use vancomycin 60 mg/kg/day IV div q6h plus cefotaxime or cefrtriaxone (as above) OR (for susceptible strains) Penicillin G 250,000 u/kg/day IV div q4h x 10 days	Some of pneumococci relatively resistant ("insensitive") or frankly resistant to penicillin and to cephalosporins
- Meningococcus (including meningococcemia)	Penicillin G 250,000 u/kg/day IV div q4h x 7 days; Regimens given for *Haemophilus* are effective for meningococcal infection; Rare strains are resistant to penicillin	Meningococcal prophylaxis: rifampin 10 mg/kg PO q12h x 4 doses; OR ceftriaxone 125-250 mg IM once; OR ciprofloxacin 500 mg PO once (adults)
- Unknown bacterial	Vancomycin AND cefotaxime or ceftriaxone (as above)	Other approved drugs: ceftazidime, ceftizoxime, meropenem
- Tuberculous	Isoniazid 15 mg/kg/day PO, IM div q12–24h AND rifampin 15 mg/kg/day, IV, PO div q12–24h x 12 mos AND streptomycin 30 mg/kg/day IM div q12h for first 4 weeks of therapy AND pyrazinamide 30 mg/kg/day PO div q12–24h for first 2 months	Hyponatremia from inappropriate ADH common; Ventricular drainage may be necessary; Steroids suppress symptoms and may improve prognosis

Clinical Diagnosis	Therapy	Comments
Shunt infections		
- *S. epidermidis* or *S. aureus*	Vancomycin 60 mg/kg/day IV div q6h OR nafcillin 150-200 mg/kg/day (?) PLUS an aminoglycoside or rifampin; x 10–14 days	Surgery for shunt revision usually necessary; May be synergy between antibiotics
- Coliform bacilli	Cefotaxime 200 mg/kg/day IV div q6h OR ampicillin 200-400 mg/kg/day IV div q6h AND gentamicin 6–7.5 mg/kg/day or amikacin 15–20 mg/kg/day IV, IM div q8h; x 21 days or longer	Select appropriate drug based on *in vitro* susceptibilities
Brain abscess	Until etiology established nafcillin or vancomycin (as for meningitis) AND cefotaxime (as for meningitis) AND metronidazole 30 mg/kg/day IV, PO div q8h; x 7–10 days after surgery; Longer therapy if no surgery	Surgery; Anaerobes common; Add anti-*Pseudomonas* drug if secondary to chronic otitis; Follow abscess size with CT scans
Herpes simplex encephalitis	Acyclovir 30 mg/kg/day as 1 hr or longer IV infusion div q8h OR vidarabine 15 mg/kg as 12 hr or longer IV infusion daily x 10 days	Larger dosages and longer durations of acyclovir therapy are being tested; (See Newborn section)
Toxoplasma encephalitis	See Section VII	

K. MISCELLANEOUS SYSTEMIC INFECTIONS

Actinomycosis	Penicillin G 250,000 u/kg/day IV div q4h until improved; thereafter penicillin V 100 mg/kg/day PO div q6h x several months	Surgery as indicated; Tetracycline for penicillin-allergic
Brucellosis	Tetracycline 40 mg/kg/day PO, div q6h <u>OR</u> doxycycline 4 mg/kg IV once daily (Pts > 7 yrs); TMP 10 mg/kg-SMX 50 mg/kg/day div q12h if < 7 yrs; Rifampin (15–20 mg/kg/day div q12h) given as second drug; x 4-6 weeks	Add gentamicin 6–7.5 mg/kg/day IV, IM div q8h for the first week for serious disease
Cat-scratch disease	Supportive; aspiration of pus	Aminoglycoside, rifampin, TMP/SMX, ciprofloxacin may be effective
Chickenpox/Shingles	Acyclovir 80 mg/kg/day PO div q6h x 5–7 days, when indicated (Most cases do not require therapy)	Parenteral therapy for severe cases (See Varicella-zoster, disseminated, page 40)
Ehrlichiosis (human monocytic or granulocytic)	(See Rickettsial infection, page 40)	
Febrile neutropenic patient	Nafcillin or oxacillin (or vancomycin if methicillin resistant Staph is suspected) <u>AND</u> anti-*Pseudomonas* beta-lactam <u>AND</u> aminoglycoside; <u>OR</u> anti-staphylococcal drug <u>AND</u> ceftazidime	If no response in 5–7 days and no bacterial etiology demonstrated, consider empiric antifungal therapy with amphotericin B; Dosages in Section VIII
Human immunodeficiency virus infection	Initial therapy with 2 (or more) drugs such as lamividine + zidovudine; Consult with HIV expert because new information about optimal regimens is emerging rapidly	See page 6 for prophylaxis for newborns

Infant botulism	No antibiotic or antitoxin; aminoglycosides potentiate effect of toxin; (trivalent antitoxin for food-borne or wound botulism)	ICU supportive therapy; Giving enemas to remove constipated stool and toxin is controversial
Influenza A infection	Amantadine 5 mg/kg/day (max 200 mg) PO div q12h x 7 days; Ribavirin aerosol (as for RSV infection, page 24) may be effective	Treat within 48–72 hrs of onset; Rx especially for high-risk patients
Kawasaki syndrome	No antibiotics; IV gamma globulin 2 g/kg as single dose	Aspirin qs to achieve serum conc of 20–30 mg/dl in acute phase; prolonged low dosage (3–5 mg/kg/day) aspirin Rx may decrease risk of coronary artery disease
Leprosy	Dapsone 100 mg PO and clofazimine 50 mg PO daily OR rifampin 600 mg PO and clofazimine 300 mg PO monthly; x 2–6 years (adult dosages)	Consult Hansen's Disease Center, Carville CA (800-642-2477) for advice about treatment
Leptospirosis	Penicillin G 250,000 u/kg/day IV, IM div q4–6h OR tetracycline 40 mg/kg/day PO div q6h; x 7–10 days	
Lyme disease	Early disease: Doxycycline 4 mg/kg/day PO div q12h (pts > 7 yrs) OR amoxicillin 40 mg/kg/day (max 3 g) (?) with probenecid 25 mg/kg/day (max 1500) PO div q8h; x 14-21 days	Late disease: ceftriaxone 100 (CNS) or 50 (others) mg/kg once daily IM, IV x 14–21 days
Measles	Supportive therapy; Ribavirin has been used 15 mg/kg/day IV div q8h x 10 days (double dose on 1st day); Vitamin A therapy reported to be beneficial in malnourished patients	Consider ribavirin in severe disease/compromised host (IV formulation not commercially available)

Clinical Diagnosis	Therapy	Comments
Melioidosis	Acute sepsis: Ceftazidime 120 mg/kg/day IV div q8h OR chloramphenicol 50–75 mg/kg/day IV, PO div q6h AND sulfisoxazole 120–150 mg/kg/day PO div q6h AND an aminoglycoside; x 10–14 days Chronic infection: Trimethoprim-sulfamethoxazole 8 mg TMP/kg–40 mg SMX/kg/day div q12h x several weeks	Ceftazidime more effective than conventional 3 drug therapy in one study Tetracycline for children > 7 years of age
Mycobacteriosis (Disseminated MAI disease in compromised host)	Usually treated with 4 or 5 drugs; e.g. ciprofloxacin, clofazimine, ethambutol, rifampin, amikacin, clarithromycin	See Section VIII for dosage
Nocardiosis	Sulfisoxazole 120–150 mg/kg/day PO div q6h x 6 weeks or longer; For severe infection, amikacin 15–20 mg/kg/day IM, IV div q8h	Surgery when indicated; Trimethoprim-sulfamethoxazole or cycloserine as alternatives
Peritonitis		
- Primary	Penicillin G 150,000 u/kg/day IV div q4h x 7–10 days	Usually pneumococcal; Other antibiotics according to culture and susceptibility tests
- Secondary to bowel perforation or appendicitis	Meropenem 60 mg/kg/day IV div q8h OR clindamycin 30 mg/kg/day IV, IM div q6h plus gentamicin 6–7.5 mg/kg/day IV, IM div q8h x 10 days or longer	Many other regimens claimed to be effective; Add ampicillin for enterococcus
- Secondary to peritoneal dialysis	Antibiotic added to dialysate in concentrations approximating those attained in serum for systemic disease (e.g. 8 mcg/ml for gentamicin; 50 mcg/ml for vancomycin, etc.)	Selection of antibiotic based on organism isolated from peritoneal fluid; Systemic antibiotics if there is accompanying bacteremia

Clinical Diagnosis	Therapy	Comments
Rickettsial infection	Tetracycline (Pts > 7 yrs) 40 mg/kg/day PO div q6h OR chloramphenicol 50–75 mg/kg/day IV div q6h; x 10–14 days	Chloramphenicol is preferred for young children
Tetanus	Metronidazole 30 mg/kg/day IV, PO div q6h OR penicillin G 100,000 u/kg/day IV div q4–6h; x 10 days	Plus antitoxin and sedation
Toxic shock syndrome	Nafcillin or oxacillin 150 mg/kg/day IV div q6h x 7 days	General supportive care of prime importance
Tularemia	Gentamicin 6–7.5 mg/kg/day IM, IV div q8h OR streptomycin 30 mg/kg/day IM div q12h; x 7–10 days (Dosage of streptomycin may be recuced by 1/2 after 3 days)	Tetracycline less effective alternative
Typhoid fever	Chloramphenicol 50–75 IV mg/kg/day div q6h OR amoxicillin 100 mg/kg/day PO div q8h x 14 days	TMP/SMX; Ceftriaxone and cefotaxime are also effective
Varicella-zoster, disseminated (compromised host)	Acyclovir 1500 mg/m^2/day (approx 45 mg/kg/day) IV as 1–2 hr infusion div q8h OR vidarabine 10 mg/kg/day as 6 hr IV infusion; x 5 days	Also used for severe or complicated chickenpox in normal host; Alternatives: famciclovir, foscarnet are more expensive

V. PREFERRED THERAPY FOR SPECIFIC BACTERIAL AND VIRAL PATHOGENS

NOTES:
1. For fungal and parasitic infections see Sections VI and VII, respectively.
2. Limitations of space do not permit listing of all possible alternative antimicrobials.

Organism	Clinical Illness	Drug of Choice	Alternatives
Acinetobacter baumanii	Sepsis, meningitis	Imipenem	Anti-*Pseudomonas* beta-lactam + amikacin; TMP/SMX
Actinobacillus actinomycetemcomitans	Abscesses, endocarditis	Ampicillin	Tetracycline (Pts > 7 yrs); chloramphenicol
Actinomyces israelii	Actinomycosis	Penicillin G	Tetracycline (Pts > 7 yrs); ampicillin; clindamycin
Aeromonas spp.	Diarrhea, sepsis, cellulitis	TMP/SMX	An aminoglycoside; imipenem
Afipia felis	Possibly, some cases of cat-scratch disease	(?) Aminoglycoside	(?) Rifampin; ciprofloxacin
Arcanobacterium haemolyticum	Pharyngitis	A macrolide	Penicillin G; a cephalosporin
Bacillus anthracis	Anthrax	Penicillin G	A macrolide; tetracycline (Pts > 7 yrs)
Bacillus cereus or *subtilis*	Sepsis	Vancomycin	Clindamycin
Bacteroides fragilis	Peritonitis, sepsis, abscesses	Chloramphenicol; clindamycin; metronidazole for CNS infection	Cefoxitin; anti-*Pseudomonas* penicillins; imipenem; meropenem

Bacteroides, other spp.	Pneumonia, sepsis, abscesses	Penicillin G or ampicillin	Clindamycin; chloramphenicol; metronidazole
Bartonella bacilliformis	Bartonellosis	Chloramphenicol; tetracycline (Pts > 7 yrs)	Penicillin G
Bartonella henselae	Cat-scratch disease	TMP/SMX; gentamicin	Rifampin; ciprofloxacin
	Bacillary angiomatosis, peliosis hepatis	A macrolide	Tetracycline (Pts > 7 yrs)
Bordetella holmesii	Sepsis	Ceftriaxone	Unknown
Bordetella pertussis, parapertussis	Pertussis	A macrolide	TMP/SMX; ampicillin
Borrelia spp.	Relapsing fever, Lyme disease	Tetracycline (Pts > 7 yrs)	Penicillin G; a cephalosporin; a macrolide
Brucella spp.	Brucellosis	Tetracycline (Pts > 7 yrs); + gentamicin	TMP/SMX; rifampin
Burkholderia cepacia	Pneumonia, sepsis	TMP/SMX	Ceftazidime; chloramphenicol
Calymmatobacterium granulomatis	Granuloma inguinale	Tetracycline (Pts > 7 yrs)	Erythromycin; TMP/SMX; an aminoglycoside
Campylobacter spp.	Diarrhea	A macrolide	Tetracycline (Pts > 7 yrs);
	Sepsis, meningitis	An aminoglycoside	According to *in vitro* tests

Organism	Clinical Illness	Drug of Choice	Alternatives
Capnocytophaga canimorsus	Sepsis following dog bite	Penicillin G	A macrolide; a cephalosporin
Capnocytophaga *ochraceae*	Sepsis, abscesses	Clindamycin	A macrolide; imipenem
Chlamydia pneumoniae (TWAR)	Pneumonia	Tetracycline (Pts > 7 yrs)	A macrolide
Chlamydia psittaci	Psittacosis	Tetracycline (Pts > 7 yrs)	Chloramphenicol
Chlamydia trachomatis	Lymphogranuloma venereum	Tetracycline (Pts > 7 yrs)	A macrolide; erythromycin
	Urethritis, vaginitis	Tetracycline or azithromycin (Pts > 7 yrs)	Erythromycin; sulfonamide; ampicillin
	Inclusion conjunctivitis of newborn	Erythromycin (oral)	Topical erythromycin, tetracycline or sulfonamide
	Pneumonia in infancy	A macrolide	Ampicillin; sulfonamide
	Trachoma	Topical + oral tetracycline (Pts > 7 yrs)	Topical + oral sulfonamide; azithromycin
Chromobacterium violaceum	Sepsis, pneumonia, abscesses	Chloramphenicol	None
Citrobacter spp.	Meningitis, sepsis	An aminoglycoside	A cephalosporin; TMP/SMX

Clostridium spp.	Tetanus, gas gangrene, sepsis	Metronidazole (+ antitoxin for tetanus)	Penicillin G; tetracycline (Pts > 7 yrs); clindamycin
Clostridium difficile	Antibiotic-associated colitis	Metronidazole (oral)	Vancomycin (oral) for metronidazole failures
Corynebacterium diphtheriae	Diphtheria	Erythromycin (+ antitoxin)	Penicillin G
Corynebacterium, JK group	Sepsis	Vancomycin	Penicillin G + gentamicin; a macrolide
Corynebacterium minutissimum	Erythrasma	Topical miconazole or clindamycin	A macrolide
Coxiella burnetii	Q fever	(See *Rickettsia*)	
Cytomegalovirus	Pneumonia, hepatitis	Ganciclovir	Foscarnet
Ehrlichia chafeensis	Human monocytic ehrlichiosis	Tetracycline (Pts > 7 yrs)	Chloramphenicol
Ehrlichia (unknown species)	Human granulocytic ehrlichiosis	Tetracycline	(?) Rifampin
Eikenella corrodens	Abscesses, meningitis	Tetracycline (Pts > 7 yrs)	Ampicillin; a macrolide; ceftriaxone

Organism	Clinical Illness	Drug of Choice	Alternatives
Enterobacter spp.	Sepsis, pneumonia, wound infection	Meropenem; imipenem	An aminoglycoside; a cephalosporin; TMP/SMX
	Urinary infection	TMP/SMX	An aminoglycoside; nitrofurantoin
Enterococcus spp.	Endocarditis, urinary infection	Ampicillin + an aminoglycoside	Vancomycin + an aminoglycoside
	NOTE: For vancomycin-resistant enterococci, consult an Infectious Disease expert.		
Erysipelothrix *insidiosa*	Sepsis, cellulitis, abscesses	Ampicillin (?) plus aminoglycoside	Tetracycline (Pts > 7 yrs)
Escherichia coli	Urinary infection, not hospital acquired	A cephalosporin	Ampicillin; amoxicillin; TMP/SMX
	Sepsis, meningitis, pneumonia, hospital acquired urinary infection	An aminoglycoside; a cephalosporin	TMP/SMX; imipenem; meropenem
Flavobacterium meningosepticum	Sepsis, meningitis	Vancomycin plus rifampin	An aminoglycoside; TMP/SMX
Francisella tularensis	Tularemia	Gentamicin or streptomycin	Tetracycline (Pts > 7 yrs); chloramphenicol
Fusobacterium spp.	Sepsis, soft tissue infection	Penicillin G	Metronidazole; clindamycin; chloramphenicol
Gardnerella vaginalis	Bacterial vaginosis	Metronidazole	Clindamycin

Haemophilus aphrophilus	Sepsis, endocarditis, abscesses	Tetracycline (Pts > 7 yrs)	Ampicillin
Haemophilus ducreyi	Chancroid or a macrolide	Ceftriaxone or a macrolide	Ciprofloxacin
Haemophilus influenzae	Upper respiratory infections	Augmentin; erythromycin-sulfa; azithromycin; clarithromycin; oral cephalosporins; TMP/SMX	Amoxicillin (if beta-lactamase negative)
	Meningitis, arthritis, cellulitis, epiglottitis, pneumonia	Cefotaxime; ceftriaxone	Ampicillin (if beta-lactamase negative); chloramphenicol
Helicobacter pylori	Gastritis, peptic ulcer	Amoxicillin (or tetracycline, Pts > 7 yrs) + metronidazole + Pepto-Bismol	Other regimens include omeprazole and clarithromycin
Herpes simplex virus	Keratoconjunctivitis	Trifluridine (topical)	Vidarabine (topical)
	Mucocutaneous	Acyclovir	None
	Encephalitis, disseminated disease	Acyclovir	Vidarabine
Human immunodeficiency virus	AIDS, ARC	Zidovudine	Didanosine; zalcitabine; stavudine
Influenza A virus	Influenza	Amantadine	(?) Ribavirin

Organism	Clinical Illness	Drug of Choice	Alternatives
Klebsiella spp.	Urinary tract infection	A cephalosporin	TMP/SMX; nitrofurantoin
	Sepsis, pneumonia, meningitis	Ceftriaxone; cefotaxime	An aminoglycoside; TMP/SMX; imipenem; meropenem
Kingella spp.	Osteomyelitis, arthritis	Ampicillin	Other beta-lactams
Legionella spp.	Legionnaires' disease and related illnesses	A macrolide + rifampin	TMP/SMX; ciprofloxacin
Leptospira spp.	Leptospirosis	Penicillin G	Tetracycline (Pts > 7 yrs)
Leptotrichia buccalis	Vincent's angina	Penicillin G	Clindamycin; tetracycline (Pts > 7 yrs); a macrolide
Listeria monocytogenes	Sepsis, meningitis	Ampicillin (?) plus aminoglycoside	TMP/SMX; vancomycin
Moraxella catarrhalis	Otitis, sinusitis, bronchitis	Augmentin; a macrolide	TMP/SMX; a cephalosporin
Moraxella other spp.	Bone and joint infection; abscess	Penicillin G	Ampicillin; an aminoglycoside
Morganella morganii	Urinary infection, sepsis	An aminoglycoside	A cephalosporin
Mycobacterium tuberculosis	Tuberculosis	Isoniazid + rifampin + pyrazinamide (? + ethambutol or streptomycin)	An aminoglycoside; cycloserine; ethionamide

Mycobacteria, nontuberculous ("atypical")	Cervical adenitis	None (surgery)	Rifampin; clarithromycin
	Other diseases	Clarithromycin or azithromycin; rifabutin; ciprofloxacin (multiple drug therapy)	amikacin; clofazimine; ethambutol
Mycobacterium marinum (*M. balnei*)	Papules, pustules, cold abscesses (Swimmer's granuloma)	None (usually self-limited)	Clarithromycin; TMP/SMX; tetracycline
Mycobacterium leprae	Leprosy	Dapsone + rifampin + clofazimine	Clarithromycin; sparfloxacin; minocycline
Mycoplasma hominis	Non-gonococcal urethritis	Clindamycin	Tetracycline (Pts > 7 yrs)
Mycoplasma pneumoniae	Pneumonia	A macrolide	Tetracycline (Pts > 7 yrs)
Neisseria gonorrhoeae	Gonorrhea	Ceftriaxone or cefixime	Spectinomycin; penicillin G (if susceptible)
Neisseria meningitidis	Sepsis, meningitis	Penicillin G or ampicillin	A cephalosporin; chloramphenicol; a sulfonamide (if susceptible)
Nocardia asteroides	Nocardiosis	A sulfonamide (+ amikacin initially)	Amikacin; TMP/SMX; cycloserine; tetracycline

Organism	Clinical Illness	Drug of Choice	Alternatives
Pasteurella multocida	Sepsis, abscesses	Penicillin G or ampicillin	Tetracycline (Pts > 7 yrs); a cephalosporin
Peptostreptococcus	Sepsis	Penicillin G or ampicillin	Clindamycin; vancomycin
Plesiomonas shigelloides	Diarrhea, meningitis	TMP/SMX	An aminoglycoside
Propionibacterium acnes	Sepsis, skin lesions	Penicillin G	Tetracycline; clindamycin; a macrolide; cephalosporin
Proteus mirabilis	Urinary infection, sepsis, meningitis	Ampicillin	An aminoglycoside; TMP/SMX; cephalosporin
Proteus, other spp.	Urinary infection, sepsis, meningitis	Cefotaxime; ceftriaxone	Imipenem; meropenem; an aminoglycoside
Providencia spp.	Sepsis	Cefotaxime; ceftriaxone	TMP/SMX; imipenem; meropenem; an aminoglycoside
Pseudomonas aeruginosa	Urinary infection	Anti-*Pseudomonas* beta-lactam	An aminoglycoside; imipenem; meropenem
	Sepsis, pneumonia	Anti-*Pseudomonas* beta-lactam + an aminoglycoside	Imipenem; meropenem; ciprofloxacin
Pseudomonas cepacia	See *Burkholderia*		
Pseudomonas mallei	Glanders	Tetracycline (Pts > 7 yrs) + streptomycin	Chloramphenicol; gentamicin

Pseudomonas pseudomallei	Melioidosis	Ceftazidime <u>OR</u> chloramphenicol + sulfa + aminoglycoside for sepsis	TMP/SMX or tetracycline (Pts > 7 yrs) for chronic disease
Respiratory syncytial virus	Bronchiolitis, pneumonia	Ribavirin	None
Rhodococcus equi	Necrotizing pneumonia	Vancomycin	An aminoglycoside; a macrolide; chloramphenicol
Rickettsia	Rocky Mountain spotted fever, Q fever, typhus, rickettsialpox	Tetracycline (Pts > 7 years)	Chloramphenicol; ciprofloxacin
Rochalimaea henselae	See *Bartonella*		
Salmonella spp.	Focal infections, typhoid fever, sepsis	Ceftriaxone; cefotaxime	TMP/SMX; chloramphenicol; ampicillin (if susceptible)
Serratia marcescens	Sepsis, pneumonia	Ceftriaxone; cefotaxime	TMP/SMX; an aminoglycoside; imipenem; meropenem
Shigella spp.	Enteritis, urinary infection, vaginitis	Ciprofloxacin	TMP/SMX; ampicillin; ceftriaxone; cefixime
Spirillum minus	Rat bite fever (sodoku)	Penicillin G or ampicillin	Tetracycline (Pts > 7 yrs); an aminoglycoside

Organism	Clinical Illness	Drug of Choice	Alternatives
Staphylococcus aureus	Skin infections	Cefadroxil; other oral cephalosporins	Cloxacillin; a macrolide; Augmentin
	Pneumonia, sepsis, osteomyelitis, etc.	Oxacillin or nafcillin	A cephalosporin; vancomycin; clindamycin
	Methicillin-resistant strains	Vancomycin (? + rifampin or aminoglycoside)	TMP/SMX; ciprofloxacin
Staphylococcus, coagulase negative	Sepsis, infected CNS shunts, urinary infection	Vancomycin	If susceptible: nafcillin (or related drug); (?) TMP/SMX
Staphylococcus spp., methicillin-resistant	Sepsis, focal infections	Vancomycin (?) + rifampin and/or gentamicin	TMP/SMX; ciprofloxacin
Stenotrophomonas maltophilia	Sepsis	TMP/SMX	Ceftazidime; ciprofloxacin
Streptobacillus moniliformis	Rat bite fever (Haverhill fever)	Penicillin G or ampicillin	Tetracycline (Pts > 7 yrs); an aminoglycoside
Streptococcus, Groups A, B, C, and G, anaerobic	Pharyngitis, impetigo, adenitis	Penicillin V or benzathine penicillin	A macrolide; a cephalosporin; clindamycin
	Pneumonia, sepsis, meningitis	Penicillin G or ampicillin	A cephalosporin; vancomycin
Streptococcus, viridans group	Endocarditis	Penicillin G + gentamicin	Vancomycin; a cephalosporin

Streptococcus pneumoniae	Pneumonia, otitis, sinusitis	Penicillin V or G; amoxicillin	A macrolide; a cephalosporin
	Meningitis, arthritis, sepsis	Penicillin G or amoxicillin	Vancomycin (for penicillin-resistant strains); cefotaxime or ceftriaxone for relatively resistant strains
Treponema pallidum	Syphilis	Penicillin G	Tetracycline (Pts > 7 yrs); ceftriaxone
Treponema pertenue	Yaws	Penicillin G	Tetracycline (Pts > 7 yrs)
Ureaplasma urealyticum	Genitourinary infections	A macrolide	Tetracycline (Pts > 7 yrs)
Varicella-zoster virus	Disseminated disease; zoster (shingles)	Acyclovir	Vidarabine; foscarnet
Vibrio cholerae	Cholera	Tetracycline (Pts > 7 yrs)	TMP/SMX; ciprofloxacin
Vibrio vulnificus	Sepsis	Tetracycline (Pts > 7 yrs)	A cephalosporin
Xanthomonas sp.	See *Stenotrophomonas*		
Yersinia enterocolitica	Enteritis, arthritis, sepsis	(?) Tetracycline (Pts > 7 yrs); TMP/SMX	A macrolide; an aminoglycoside
Yersinia pestis	Plague	Streptomycin + chloramphenicol or tetracycline (Pts > 7 yrs)	Other aminoglycoside
Yersinia pseudotuberculosis	Adenitis	(?) Tetracycline	(?) TMP/SMX

VI. ANTIFUNGAL THERAPY

Infection	Therapy	Comments
SYSTEMIC INFECTIONS		
Aspergillosis	Amphotericin B 1.0 mg/kg IV daily as 3-4 hour infusion in 5% dextrose sol'n (no saline); Total dosage 30–35 mg/kg given over period of 6 weeks or longer; For patients not tolerating or failing to respond, Abelcet 5 mg/kg IV daily or Amphotec 3-5 mg/kg daily can be used; Itraconazole may be considered for indolent, non-CNS disease (For allergic broncho-pulmonary aspergillosis, see page 28)	Treat for tissue invasion, not colonization; Monitor K, Mg, HCO_3, Hgb and renal function; Azotemia common; Sodium loading may help azotemia; Total dosage and duration of therapy individualized
Blastomycosis (North American)	Itraconazole 200–400 mg/day (adults), (?) 4 mg/kg/day (pediatric dosage not established) PO OR amphotericin B (as above) for severe disease; x 6 months	Alternative: ketoconazole 6 mg/kg/day PO div q12–24 hr
Candidiasis		
- Disseminated infection	Amphotericin B (as above) but daily dosage 0.5–0.75 mg/kg OR amphotericin B PLUS flucytosine 100 mg/kg/day PO div q6h; OR Albelcet (as above); Fluconazole 6-12 mg/kg IV or PO daily for noncompromized host	Hematologic toxicity and diarrhea with flucytosine; Keep serum conc <100 mcg/ml; Replace IV catheter in catheter-associated candidemia
- Urinary infection	Fluconazole 3–6 mg/kg once daily OR flucytosine 50 mg/kg/day div q6h; Amphotericin B (50 mcg/ml) bladder irrigation if catheter in place	Stopping antibiotic or removing Foley catheter sometimes leads to spontaneous cure in the normal host

- Oropharyngeal, esophageal	Clotrimazole 10 mg troche PO 5 x daily x 7 days OR fluconazole 3 mg/kg once daily OR itraconazole oral sol'n 10-20 ml (adult dose) squished in mouth and swallowed once daily OR amphotericin B suspension 1 ml qid	Amphotericin B for severe disease or febrile neutropenic pts; Miconazole gel (not available in U.S.) best for thrush in infants
Chromomycosis	Flucytosine OR itraconazole (as above)	
Coccidioidomycosis	Amphotericin B (as above) for severe, non-CNS disease OR (for non-life threatening disease) itraconazole 200 mg bid PO (adult dose) OR fluconazole 6-12 mg/kg once daily for meningitis	Consider intrathecal amphotericin B for fluconazole failures in meningitis
Cryptococcosis	Amphotericin B 0.7 mg/kg IV daily +/- flucytosine 100 mg/kg/day PO div q6h; Monitor flucytosine serum concentrations	For HIV-positive, amph B x 2 wks, then fluconazole 6-12 mg/kg once daily for 10 wks, then 4 mg/kg daily indefinitely
Histoplasmosis	Amphotericin B 0.5 mg/kg IV daily OR (for non-life threatening disease) itraconazole 200 mg b.i.d. PO (adults)	Ketoconazole (as above) as alternative
Mucormycosis (zygomycosis)	Amphotericin B (as for aspergillosis) x 6 wks or longer	Surgery, as necessary; Control of diabetes mellitus, if present
Paracoccidioidomycosis	Itraconazole 100 mg/day PO (adult OR amphotericin B (as for aspergillosis)	Ketoconazole (as above) as alternative; Sulfa drugs less effective but inexpensive

Infection	Therapy	Comments
Phaeohyphomycosis	Amphotericin B (as for aspergillosis) x 3 wks or longer	Surgery, as necessary; Itraconazole (as above) for indolent, non-CNS disease may be useful
***Pneumocystis carinii* pneumonia**	Trimethoprim-sulfamethoxazole 15–20 mg TMP–75–100 mg SMX/kg/day IV, PO div q6h OR pentamidine isethionate 4 mg base/kg/day IV daily x 10–14 days; Alternatives: trimethoprim and dapsone; primaquine and clindamycin; trimetrexate and folinic acid; atovaquone for non-severe disease	Prophylaxis: 5 mg TMP–25 mg SMX/kg/day PO div q12 q12–24 hr given daily or 3 times weekly; 2 mg/kg/day PO OR 300 mg aerosolized pentamidine monthly
***Pseudallescheria boydii* and *Scedosporium apiospermum* infection**	Miconazole 20–40 mg/kg/day IV div q8h x 3 weeks or longer	Ketoconazole or itraconazole may be effective
Sporotrichosis	Itraconazole 100–200 mg/day PO (adult dosage); amphotericin B (as for aspergillosis) or itraconazole 200 mg b.i.d. for extracutaneous disease	Alternative: Saturated sol'n of potassium iodide 1-2 drops per year of age 3 x daily PO (maximum 30 drops t.i.d.) until lymphocutaneous lesions resolved (give with fruit juice or milk)
LOCALIZED MUCOCUTANEOUS INFECTIONS		
Dermatophytoses		
- Scalp (including kerion)	Griseofulvin ultramicronized 10 mg/kg or micronized 15 mg/kg once daily x 1–2 mos or longer (taken with milk or fatty foods to augment absorption) OR ketoconazole 6 mg/kg/day div q12–24h; Itraconazole or	Topical antifungal agent may prevent recurrence from endothrix spores; Selenium sulfide shampoo twice weekly may be useful adjunct

- Glabrous skin, hands or feet	Topical butenafine, ciclopirox, clotrimazole, econazole, ketoconazole, miconazole, naftifine, sulconazole, terbinafine and tolnaftate equally effective; Apply 2 x daily x 7-10 days	Undecylemic acid less effective; Longer treatment needed for palmar/plantar infection; Keep toe webs and groin dry; Treat bacterial superinfection
- Tinea versicolor *[Pityrosporum ovale (Malassezia furfur)]*	Selenium sulfide (Selsun) <u>OR</u> topical clotrimazole (or related drug) applied twice daily x 7–10 days	Recurrence common; Itraconazole useful for extensive lesions
- Tinea unguium (Onychomycosis)	Itraconazole 200 mg bid PO or terbinafine 500 mg daily (adult doses) for 1 week per month x 3 months (hands) or 6 months (toes) until new nail growth	Recurrence or partial response common
Candidiasis		
- Benign mucocutaneous	Topical ketoconazole, econazole, nystatin, clotrimazole or miconazole 3–4 x daily x 7–10 days	0.5% aqueous gentian violet for refractory cases
- Oropharyngeal, esophageal	(See above)	
- Chronic mucocutaneous	Itraconazole 200 mg PO daily (adult dosage) <u>OR</u> fluconazole 3 mg/kg daily PO until lesions clear	Occurs in hosts with variety of immune defects
- Vulvovaginal	Vaginal cream with butoconazole, clotrimazole, miconazole, terconazole or tioconazole; <u>OR</u> vaginal tablets/suppositories of clotrimazole, miconazole, terconazole; all at bedtime x 3–7 days; <u>OR</u> single 4-5 mg/kg dose of fluconazole	Avoid fluconazole in pregnancy

VII. ANTIPARASITIC THERAPY

Note: Familiarize yourself with the toxic potentials of these drugs and monitor the patient accordingly. For some of the parasitic diseases, drugs available only from the Centers for Disease Control are the preferred therapy; these drugs are indicated by "(CDC)." Consultation for diagnostic tests and detailed information about experimental drugs are available from the CDC and they will send drugs to you. The telephone number is 1-770-488-7788.

Disease/Organism	Treatment
AMEBIASIS *Entamoeba histolytica*	
- Asymptomatic carrier	Iodoquinol (formerly diiodohydroxyquin) 30-40 mg/kg/day (max 2 g) PO div q8h x 20 days OR paromomycin 30 mg/kg/day PO div q8h x 7–10 days OR diloxanide furoate (CDC) 20 mg/kg/day PO div q8h x 10 days
- Mild to moderate colitis	Metronidazole 35–50 mg/kg/day PO div q8h x 10 days OR tinidazole 50 mg/kg/day (max 2 g) x 3 days OR paromomycin 30 mg/kg/day PO div q8h x 7–10 days; FOLLOWED BY iodoquinol, as above, x 20 days
- Severe colitis, liver abscess	Metronidazole 35–50 mg/kg/day PO, IV div q8h x 10 days FOLLOWED BY iodoquinol or paromomycin, as above
AMEBIC MENINGOENCEPHALITIS *Naegleria* spp., *Acanthamoeba* spp., *Hartmannella* spp.	Amphotericin B 1 mg/kg/day IV x (?) 3-4 weeks, (?) PLUS miconazole and rifampin for *Naegleria*; Intrathecal miconazole (10 mg) daily may be helpful; *Acanthamoeba* susceptible *in vitro* to ketoconazole, flucytosine, pentamidine

Disease / Organism	Treatment
Ancylostoma duodenale	See HOOKWORM
ANGIOSTRONGYLIASIS *Angiostrongylus* spp.	Thiabendazole 50–75 mg/kg/day (max 3g) PO div q8h for *A. costaricensis* x 3 days OR mebendazole 100 mg PO b.i.d. x 5 days for *A. cantonensis*
ANISAKIASIS *Anasakis* spp.	Removal by fibroendoscopy or surgery
ASCARIASIS *Ascaris lumbricoides*	Mebendazole 100 mg b.i.d. x 3 days OR albendazole 400 mg, one dose OR pyrantel pamoate 11 mg/kg (max 1 g), one dose
BABESIOSIS *Babesia* spp.	Clindamycin (30 mg/kg/day PO div q8h) PLUS quinine (25 mg/kg/day PO div q8h) x 7 days effective in limited experience; Exchange blood transfusion reported helpful; atovaquone plus azithromycin may be effective
BALANTIDIASIS *Balantidium coli*	Metronidazole 35–50 mg/kg/day PO div q8h x 5 days OR tetracycline (Pts >7 yrs) 40 mg/kg/day PO div q6h x 10 days OR iodoquinol 40 mg/kg/day (max 2 g/day) PO div q8h x 20 days
BLASTOCYSTIASIS *Blastocystis hominis*	Metronidazole 35–50 mg/kg/day PO div q8h x 10 days OR iodoquinol 40 mg/kg/day (max 2 g) PO div q8h x 20 days (Need for treatment is controversial)
CAPILLARIASIS *Capillaria philippinensis*	Mebendazole or albendazole 200 mg PO b.i.d. x 10-20 days OR thiabendazole 25 mg/kg/day (max 3 gm) PO div q12h x 30 days
CHAGA'S DISEASE *Trypanosoma cruzi*	See TRYPANOSOMIASIS

Disease/Organism	Treatment
Clonorchis sinensis	See FLUKES
CRYPTOSPORIDIOSIS *Cryptosporidium parvum*	No proven effective therapy; Paromomycin or azithromycin may be effective
CUTANEOUS LARVA MIGRANS or CREEPING ERUPTION (Cutaneous hookworm)	Thiabendazole suspension topically b.i.d. x 2–5 days; OR ivermectin 200 mcg/kg PO, one dose; OR albendazole 200 mg bid PO x 3 days; OR thiabendazole 50 mg/kg/day (max 3 g) PO div q12h x 3 days; Note: ethylene chloride spray and carbon dioxide snow are effective but painful and sometimes damage tissue
CYCLOSPORIASIS *Cyclospora* sp. (Cyanobacterium-like agent)	Trimethoprim-sulfamethoxazole (10 mg TMP–50 mg SMX/kg/day) PO div q12h x 5-7 days
CYSTICERCOSIS *Cysticercus cellulosae*	Albendazole 15 mg/kg/day PO div q12h (max 800 mg/day) x 8-30 days OR praziquantel 50 mg/kg/day PO div q8h x 14 days; For CNS cysticercosis give steroids before first dose; Steroids can affect metabolism of albendazole and praziquantel (Therapy for active lesions only)
DIENTAMEBIASIS *Dientamoeba fragilis*	Iodoquinol 40 mg/kg/day (max 2 g) PO div q8h x 20 days OR tetracycline (Pts > 7 yr) 40 mg/kg/day PO div q6h x 7–10 days OR paromomycin 25 mg/kg/day div q8h x 7 days
Diphyllobothrium latum	See TAPEWORMS
DIROFILARIASIS *Dirofilaria immitis*	Surgical excision of subcutaneous or pulmonary nodules; Albendazole possibly effective
DRACUNCULIASIS *Dracunculus medinensis* (Guinea worm)	Metronidazole 25 mg/kg/day PO div q8h x 10 days OR thiabendazole 50–75 mg/kg PO div q12h x 3 days (not curative but reduces inflammation); IN ADDITION remove worm by winding out a few cm each day; Mebendazole 400-800 mg/day PO x 6 days may be curative

Infection	Treatment
ECHINOCOCCOSIS *Echinococcus granulosus*	Surgical treatment when indicated; Albendazole 15 mg/kg/day PO div q12h x 28 days followed by 14 days without drug; give 3 cycles of therapy
Entamoeba histolytica	See AMEBIASIS
Enterobius vermicularis	See PINWORMS
Fasciola hepatica	See FLUKES
FILARIASIS	
- River blindness *Onchocerca volvulus*	Ivermectin 150 mcg/kg PO, one dose; Repeat q6–12mos; Antihistamines or corticosteroids for allergic reactions
- Other forms (loa loa, tropical eosinophilia) *Wuchereria bancrofti, Brugia malayi*	Diethylcarbamazine 1 mg/kg on Day 1, 1 mg/kg t.i.d. on Day 2, 2 mg/kg t.i.d. on Day 3; then 6 mg/kg/day (9 mg/kg/day for loa loa) PO div q8h x 18 days; Antihistamines or corticosteroids for allergic reactions; Surgical excision of subcutaneous nodules, preferably before drug therapy; Ivermectin may be effective; NOTE: In heavy infections consider giving albendazole or ivermectin initially to reduce counts before diethylcarbamazine therapy in loa loa
FLUKES	
- Sheep liver fluke (*Fasciola hepatica*) - Lung fluke (*Paragonimus westermani*) - Chinese liver fluke (*Clonorchis sinensis*) and others (*Fasciolopsis, Heterophyes, Metagonimus, Opisthorchis*)	Praziquantel 75 mg/kg PO div q8h x 1 day (x 2 days for *P. westermani*) is the drug of choice for all fluke infections except *F. hepatica* for which bithionol (CDC) is given (30–50 mg/kg PO div q.i.d. on alternate days x 10–15 doses)

Disease/Organism	Treatment
GIARDIASIS *Giardia lamblia*	Furazolidone 6–8 mg/kg/day PO div q6h x 7–10 days OR metronidazole 15 mg/kg/day PO div q8h x 5 days; Quinacrine effective but not easily available in the U.S. (All can have Antabuse-like effect)
GNATHOSTOMIASIS *Gnathostoma spinigerum*	Surgical removal PLUS albendazole 15 mg/kg/day x 21 days; Ivermectin may be effective
HOOKWORM *Necator americanus*, *Ancylostoma duodenale*	Mebendazole 100 mg PO b.i.d. x 3 days OR pyrantel pamoate 11 mg/kg (max 1 g/day) PO daily x 3 days; OR albendazole 10 mg/kg (max 400 mg), one dose
Hymenolepis nana	See TAPEWORMS
ISOSPORIASIS *Isospora belli*	Trimethoprim-sulfamethoxazole 10 mg TMP–50 mg SMX/kg/day div q6h x 10 days; Then, 5 mg TMP–25 mg SMX/kg/day PO div q12h x 3 wks; Pyrimethamine may be effective
LEISHMANIASIS, including kala azar *Leishmania braziliensis*, *L. donovani, L. tropica, L. mexicana*	Stibogluconate sodium (CDC) 20 mg/kg/day (max 800 mg) IM or IV, daily x 20-28 days (10 mg/kg/day x 10 days for *L. tropica*); ALTERNATIVES, pentamidine isethionate 4 mg/kg/day IM daily for 14 days OR, amphotericin B 1 mg/kg/day IV x 4–8 wks; Ketaconazole may be effective for cutaneous leishmaniasis (Concomitant treatment with interferon gamma has been used for refractory cases of visceral disease)
LICE *Pediculus capitis* or *humanus*, *Pthirus pubis*	Permethrin 1% (Nix Creme Rinse) OR pyrethins (RID, A-200 Pyrinate liquid or shampoo, R & C Shampoo) OR lindane (Kwell) applied topically once (follow manufacturer's instructions for use); Repeat in 1 wk; OR ivermectin 200 mcg/kg PO, one dose; For eyelash infestation, use petrolatum; Launder bedding and clothing

MALARIA	CDC Malaria Hotline 1-770-488-7788; It is advisable for physicians who are not familiar with treating malaria to consult with CDC physicians; The following suggestions for treatment do not cover all situations.
Prophylaxis - For areas without chloroquine-resistant *P. falciparum*	Chloroquine 5 mg base/kg (max 300 mg) PO once weekly, beginning 1 week before arrival in malarial zone and continuing for 4 weeks after last exposure (drugs available in liquid form outside the U.S.); PLUS (optional) beginning with final 2 weeks of chloroquine Rx, primaquine 0.3 mg base/kg PO daily x 14 days after departure from endemic area for individuals heavily exposed to mosquitoes
- For areas where chloroquine-resistant *P. falciparum* exists	Chloroquine (as above); Have pyrimethamine-sulfadoxine (Fansidar) available to take if febrile illness develops; OR mefloquine for children > 45 kg 250 mg once weekly starting 1 week before travel and for 4 weeks after leaving area; for children 15–19 kg, 1/4 tab; 20–30 kg, 1/2 tab; 31–45 kg, 3/4 tab OR doxycycline (Pt > 7 yr) 2 mg/kg (max 100 mg) daily
Treatment of disease - *Plasmodium vivax, P. ovale P. malariae*, chloroquine-susceptible *P. falciparum*	Chloroquine 10 mg base/kg (max 600 mg) PO stat, then 5 mg base/kg at 6 hrs, 24 hrs and 48 hrs after initial dose; For parenteral therapy, quinidine 10 mg/kg (max 600 mg) IV (1 hr infusion) followed by continuous infusion of 0.02 mg/kg/min until oral therapy can be given (3 days maximum); It is advisable to monitor patients receiving quinidine in an ICU setting; Prevention of relapse (*P. vivax, P. ovale)*: primaquine 0.3 mg base/kg/day x 14 days

(continued on next page)

Disease/Organism	Treatment
MALARIA (cont'd.)	
- *P. falciparum* chloroquine-resistant	Quinine 25 mg/kg/day (max 2 g/day) PO div q8h x 3 days (or longer) AND Fansidar (pyrimethamine-sulfadoxine): < 1 yr, 1/4 tab; 1–3 yr, 1/2 tab; 4–8 yr, 1 tab; 9–14 yr, 2 tab; > 14 yrs, 3 tab as a single dose on last day of quinine; NOTE: Several alternative regimens have been reported for Fansidar-resistant infections: Check with the CDC; For parenteral therapy, quinidine, as above; NOTE:Corticosteroids are contraindicated in cerebral malaria; Iron chelation therapy may be beneficial in cerebral malaria
Paragonimus westermani	See FLUKES
PINWORMS *Enterobius vermicularis*	Mebendazole 100 mg PO, one dose OR albendazole 400 mg PO, one dose OR pyrantel pamoate 11 mg/kg (max 1 gm) PO, one dose; Repeat treatment in 2 weeks
PNEUMOCYSTIS PNEUMONIA *Pneumocystis carinii*	See page 56
SCABIES *Sarcoptes scabei*	Permethrim 5% cream applied to entire body (including scalp in infants), left on for 8–14 hr before bathing OR lindane (Kwell) lotion applied to all of body below neck, leave on overnight, bathe in a.m. OR ivermectin 200 mcg/kg PO, one dose; Launder bedding and clothing; Topical corticosteroid after treatment for severe, persistent itching
SCHISTOSOMIASIS *Schistosoma hematobium, japonicum, mansoni, mekongi*	Praziquantel 40–60 mg/kg/day PO in 2–3 doses taken in 1 day
STRONGYLOIDIASIS *Strongyloides stercoralis*	Thiabendazole 50 mg/kg/day (max 3 g/d) PO div q12h x 2 days (5 days or longer for disseminated disease) OR invermectin 200 mcg/kg daily x 2 days

Infection	Treatment
TAPEWORMS	
- *Cysticercus cellulosae*	See CYSTICERCOSIS
- *Echinococcus granulosus*	See ECHINOCOCCOSIS
- *Taenia saginata, T. solium, Hymenolepis nana, Diphyllobothrium latum, Dipylidium caninum*	Praziquantel 5–10 mg/kg x 1 dose (25 mg/kg daily x 6 days for *H. nana*) OR niclosamide tablet approx 40 mg/kg PO chewed thoroughly x 1 dose
TOXOPLASMOSIS *Toxoplasma gondii*	Pyrimethamine 2 mg/kg/day PO div q12h x 3 days (max 100 mg) then 1 mg/kg/day (max 25 mg every day) PO (supplemental folinic acid) AND sulfadiazine 120 mg/kg/day PO div q6h (max 6 g/day) OR spiramycin (CDC) 50–100 mg/kg/day PO div q6h; Treatment continued for 4 wks after resolution of illness (See page 8 for congenital toxoplasmosis); Corticosteroids given for ocular infection; Prophylaxis: Trimethoprim-sulfamethoxazole, as for *Pneumocystis* (page 58)
TRICHINOSIS *Trichinella spiralis*	Anti-inflammatory drugs; Steroids for CNS or severe symptoms; Mebendazole 200–400 mg t.i.d. x 3 days, then 400–500 mg t.i.d. x 10 days
TRICHOMONIASIS *Trichomonas vaginalis*	Metronidazole 40 mg/kg (max 2 g) PO x 1 dose OR metronidazole 15 mg/kg/day (max 1 g/day) PO div q8h x 7 days; Treat sex partners
TRICHOSTRONGYLIASIS *Trichostrongylus orientalis*	Mebendazole 100 mg b.i.d. x 3 days OR pyrantel pamoate 11 mg/kg, one dose

Disease/Organism	Treatment
Trichuris trichiura	See WHIPWORM
TRYPANOSOMIASIS	
- **CHAGA'S DISEASE** *Trypanosoma cruzi*	Nifurtimox (CDC) or benznidazole (CDC); Obtain dosage recommendations from CDC; Gamma interferon has been added to regimen in some patients
- **SLEEPING SICKNESS** *T. brucei gambiense*; *T. brucei rhodesiense*	Acute stage: suramin (CDC) 20 mg/kg IV on Days 1, 3, 7, 14 and 21 (max 1 g) OR pentamidine isethionate 4 mg/kg/day IM x 10 days Late disease with CNS involvement: Melarsoprol (CDC) initial dose 0.36 mg/kg IV, gradually increase dosage to maximum dose of 3.6 mg/kg given at 1–5 day intervals for total of 10 doses (18–25 mg/kg) during a 1 month period For acute and CNS disease: eflornithine 400 mg/kg/day IV div q6h x 14 days, followed by 300 mg/kg/day PO x 3-4 weeks
VISCERAL LARVA MIGRANS *Toxocara canis; T. cati*	Thiabendazole 50 mg/kg/day PO div q12h x 5 days or longer OR albendazole 400 mg b.i.d. x 3-5 days OR diethylcarbamazine 6 mg/kg/day div q8h x 7–10 days; Corticosteroids for severe symptoms and for eye involvement
WHIPWORM (TRICHURIASIS) *Trichuris trichiura*	Mebendazole 100 mg PO b.i.d. x 3 days OR albendazole 400 mg PO, one dose
Wuchereria bancrofti	See FILARIASIS

VIII. ALPHABETICAL LISTING OF ANTIBIOTICS WITH DOSAGE FORMS AND USUAL DOSAGES

NOTES:
1. When a range of dosage is given, the higher dosages are generally indicated for serious illnesses.
2. In some cases the dosages indicated differ from the manufacturers' recommendations in the package inserts.
3. IV preparations available in ready-to-use "piggy-back" bottles are not included in the tabulated dosage forms.

Generic and Trade® Names	Dosage Form	Route	Dosage	Interval
Acyclovir Zovirax®, generic	500, 1000 mg vial	IV	25–50 mg/kg/day	q8h
	200 mg/5 ml susp	PO	80 mg/kg/day	q6h
	200 mg cap; 400, 800 mg tab	PO	1 cap 5 times daily; 1 tab 4 times daily	
Albendazole Albenza®	200 mg tab	PO	15 mg/kg/day	q12h
Amantadine HCl Symmetrel®, generic	100 mg cap 50 mg/5 ml syrup	PO	5–8 mg/kg/day (max 200 mg/day)	q12h
Amikacin sulfate generic	0.1, 0.2, 0.5, 1 g vials	IM, IV	15–22.5 mg/kg/day (See page 2 re q24h dosing)	q8h
Amoxicillin trihydrate Amoxil®, Wymox®, generic	250, 500 mg cap 125, 250 mg/5 ml susp 125, 250 mg chewable tab 50 mg/1 ml drops	PO	40 mg/kg/day	q8h

Amoxicillin and clavulanate potassium Augmentin®	7:1 Formulation: 875/125 mg tab 200/28.5, 400/57 mg chewable tab 200/28.5, 400/57 mg/5 ml susp	PO	7:1 Formulation: 45 mg amoxicillin component/kg/day	q12h
	4:1 Formulation: 500/125 mg tab 125/31.25, 250/62.5 mg chewable tab 125/31.25, 250/62.5 mg/5 ml susp		4:1 Formulation: 30 mg amoxicillin component/kg/day	q8h
Amphotericin B Fungizone®	50 mg vial 100 mg/ml susp	IV PO	0.25–1 mg/kg/day 4-12 ml/day	q1–2 days q6h
Amphotericin B, cholesteryl sulfate AMPHOTEC®	50, 100 mg vial	IV	3-6 mg/kg/day	q24h
Amphotericin B, liposomal ABELCET®	100 mg vial	IV	5 mg/kg/day	q24h
Ampicillin and Ampicillin trihydrate Omnipen®, generic	250, 500 mg cap 125, 250/5 ml susp 100 mg/ml drops	PO	50 mg/kg/day	q6h

Generic and Trade® Names	Dosage Form	Route	Dosage	Interval
Ampicillin, sodium Omnipen®, generic	0.125, 0.25, 0.5, 1, 2, 4 g vials	IM, IV	100–200 mg/kg/day (meningitis 200–400)	q6h
Ampicillin/Sulbactam Unasyn®	1 g amp/0.5 g sul, 2 g amp/1 g sul	IV	As per ampicillin; Not approved for children	q6h
Atovaquone Mepron®	750 mg/5 ml susp	PO	(?) 40 mg/kg/day with meals	q8h
Azithromycin Zithromax®	250 mg cap 600 mg Tab 100, 200 mg/5 ml susp	PO	Otitis/pneumonia: 10 mg/kg/day loading dose, then 5 mg/kg/day Pharyngitis: 12 mg/kg/day	q24h
Aztreonam Azactam®	0.5, 1, 2 g vials	IM, IV	90–120 mg/kg/day	q6–8h
Bacampicillin HCl Spectrobid®	400 mg tab (equivalent to 280 mg ampicillin) 125 mg/5 ml	PO	25–50 mg/kg/day	q12h
Carbenicillin indanyl sodium Geocillin®	382 mg tab	PO	30–50 mg/kg/day	q6h
Cefaclor Ceclor®, generic	125, 187, 250, 375 mg/5 ml susp 250, 500 mg cap	PO	40 mg/kg/day	q8–12h
Cefadroxil monohydrate Duricef®	500 mg cap, 1 g tab 125, 250, 500 mg/5 ml susp	PO	30 mg/kg/day	q12h

Cefamandole nafate Mandol®	0.5, 1, 2 g vials	IV, IM	100–150 mg/kg/day	q4–6h
Cefazolin sodium Ancef®, Kefzol®	0.5, 1 g vials	IM, IV	50–100 mg/kg/day	q8h
Cefepime HCl Maxipime®	1, 2 g vials	IV, IM	1-4q/day for adults (Not approved for children)	q12h
Cefixime Suprax®	200, 400 mg tab 100 mg/5 ml susp	PO	8 mg/kg/day	q12–24h
Cefonicid sodium Monocid®	0.5, 1 g vials	IV, IM	(?) 20–40 mg/kg/day (Not approved for children)	q24h
Cefoperazone sodium Cefobid®	1, 2 g vials	IV, IM	100–150 mg/kg/day (Not approved for children)	q8–12h
Cefotaxime sodium Claforan®	0.5, 1, 2 g vials	IV, IM	50–180 mg/kg/day (meningitis 300 div q6h)	q6–8h
Cefotetan disodium Cefotan®	1, 2 g vials	IV, IM	(?) 40–80 mg/kg/day (Not approved for children)	q12h
Cefoxitin sodium Mefoxin®	1, 2 g vials	IV, IM	80–160 mg/kg/day	q4–6h

Generic and Trade® Names	Dosage Form	Route	Dosage	Interval
Cefpodoxime proxetil Vantin®	100, 200 mg tab 50, 100 mg/5 ml susp	PO	10 mg/kg/day (max 400 mg)	q12h
Cefprozil Cefzil®	250, 500 mg tab 125, 250 mg/5 ml susp	PO	15 mg/kg/day (otitis 30)	q12h
Ceftazidime Ceptaz®, Fortaz®, Pentacef® Tazicef®, Tazidime®	0.5, 1, 2 g vials	IV, IM	100–150 mg/kg/day (meningitis 150)	q8h
Ceftibuten Cedax®	400 mg cap 90, 180 mg/5 ml susp	PO	9 mg/kg/day	q24h
Ceftizoxime sodium Cefizox®	1, 2 g vials	IV, IM	150–200 mg/kg/day	q6–8h
Ceftriaxone sodium Rocephin®	0.25, 0.5, 1, 2 g vials	IM, IV	50–75 mg/kg/day (meningitis 100)	q12–24h
Cefuroxime axetil Ceftin®	125, 250, 500 mg tab 125, 250 mg/5 ml susp	PO	20 mg/kg/day (30 for otitis, impetigo)	q12h
Cefuroxime sodium Kefurox®, Zinacef®	0.75, 1.5 g vials	IV, IM	100–150 mg/kg/day (meningitis 240)	q8h q6h
Cephalexin Biocef®, Keflex®, Keftab®, generic	250, 500 mg tab 0.25, 0.5, 1 g cap 100 mg/ml drops 125, 250 mg/5 ml susp	PO	25–50 mg/kg/day	q6h

Cephalothin, sodium Kefzol®, generic	1, 2, 4 g vials	IM, IV	75–125 mg/kg/day	q4–6h
Cephradine Generic	250, 500 mg cap 125, 250 mg/5 ml susp	PO	25–50 mg/kg/day	q6h
	0.25, 0.5, 1 g vials	IM, IV	50–100 mg/kg/day	q6h
Chloramphenicol sodium succinate Chloromycetin®	1 g vial	IV	50–75 mg/kg/day (meningitis 75–100)	q6h
Chloroquine HCl Aralen HCl®	250 mg amp (equiv to 200 mg base)	IM	5 mg base/kg	1 or 2 doses
Chloroquine PO_4 Aralen PO_4®, generic	500 mg tab (equiv to 300 mg base)	PO	10 mg base/kg/day	q24h
Chloroquine, hydroxy Plaquenil®	200 mg tab (equiv to 155 mg base)			
Cinoxacin generic	500 mg cap	PO	1 g/day (adult dose)	q6–12h
Ciprofloxacin Cipro®	100, 250, 500, 750 mg tab	PO	(?) 20–30 mg/kg/day (Not approved for < 18 yrs, except for cystic fibrosis)	q12h
	200, 400 mg vial	IV		

Generic and Trade® Names	Dosage Form	Route	Dosage	Interval
Clarithromycin Biaxin®	250, 500 mg tab 125, 250 mg/5 ml susp	PO	15 mg/kg/day	q12h
Clindamycin HCl	75, 150, 300 mg cap	PO	10–20 mg/kg/day	q6–8h
Clindamycin palmitate HCl	75 mg/5 ml sol'n			
Clindamycin phosphate Cleocin®, generic	0.3, 0.6, 0.9 g vials	IM, IV	20–40 mg/kg/day	q6–8h
Clofazime Lamprene®	50 mg cap	PO	100 mg/day (adult dosage)	q24h
Cloxacillin, sodium generic	250, 500 mg cap 125 mg/5 ml sol'n	PO	50–100 mg/kg/day	q6h
Colistimethate, sodium Coly-Mycin M®	150 mg vial	IM, IV	5–7 mg/kg/day	q8h
Colistin sulfate Coly-Micin S®	25 mg/5 ml susp	PO	15 mg/kg/day	q8h
Cycloserine Seromycin®	250 mg cap	PO	(?) 7–10 mg/kg/day (No established dosage for children)	q12h
Dapsone	25, 100 mg scored tab	PO	1 mg/kg/day	q24h
Demeclocycline HCl Declomycin®	150 mg cap 150, 300 mg tab	PO	8–12 mg/kg/day (Pts > 7 yrs)	q6–12h

Dicloxacillin sodium Dycill®, generic	125, 250, 500 mg cap 62.5 mg/5 ml susp	PO	12–25 mg/kg/day	q6h
Didanosine (ddI) Videx®	25, 50, 100, 150 mg chewable tab 100, 167, 250, 375 mg powder for oral solution	PO	240 mg/m^2/day	q12h
Diiodohydroxyquin (See Iodoquinol)				
Dirithromycin Dynabac®	250 mg tab	PO	500 mg (adult dosage) (Not approved for children)	q24h
Doxycycline Doryx®, Vibramycin®, Vibra-Tabs®, generic	50, 100 mg cap 100 mg tab 25 mg/5 ml susp 50 mg/5 ml syrup	PO	2–4 mg/kg/day (Pts > 7 yrs)	q12h on 1st day; then 1/2 dose q24h
	100 mg vials	IV	2–4 mg/kg/day (Pts >7 yrs)	q24h as 2-hr infusion
Enoxacin Penetrex®	200, 400 mg tab	PO	400–800 mg/day (adult dosage)	q12h

Generic and Trade® Names	Dosage Form	Route	Dosage	Interval
Erythromycin E-Mycin®, ERYC®, Ery-Tab®, Erythromycin Base Filmtab®, PCE Dispertab®, generic	125 mg pellets in cap 250 mg tab, cap 333 mg tab	PO	40 mg/kg/day	q6h
	2% topical sol'n for acne 0.5% ophthalmic ointment	Topical Topical		
Erythromycin estolate Ilosone®, generic	100 mg/ml drops 500 mg tab 125, 250 mg cap 125, 250 mg chewable tab 125, 250 mg/5 ml susp	PO	30–40 mg/kg/day	q8–12h
Erythromycin ethylsuccinate E.E.S.®, EryPed®, generic	400 mg tab 200 mg chewable tab 200, 400 mg/5 ml susp 100 mg/2.5 ml drops	PO	40 mg/kg/day	q8h
Erythromycin ethylsuccinate and sulfisoxazole acetyl Pediazole®, Eryzole®, generic	200 mg erythromycin and 600 mg sulfisoxazole/5 ml susp	PO	40 mg/kg/day of erythromycin component	q6–8h
Erythromycin gluceptate Ilotycin Gluceptate®	0.25, 0.5, 1 g amp	IV	20–50 mg/kg/day	continuous infusion or q6h
Erythromycin lactobionate	0.5, 1 g vial	IV	20–40 mg/kg/day	q6h (1–2 hr infusion)

Erythromycin stearate Erythrocin®, generic	250, 500 mg tab	PO	20–40 mg/kg/day	q6h
Ethambutol hydrocloride Myambutol®	100, 400 mg tab	PO	15 mg/kg/day	q24h
Ethionamide Trecator-SC®	250 mg tab	PO	(?) 10–20 mg/kg/day (No established dosage for children)	q12h
Famciclovir Famvir®	125, 250, 500 mg tab	PO	250 mg for herpes 1500 mg for zoster (adult dosages)	q12h q8h
Famsidar (See sulfadoxine and pyrimethamine)				
Fluconazole Diflucan®	50, 100, 200 mg tab 50, 200 mg/5 ml susp 200, 400 mg vial	PO IV	3–6 mg/kg/day	q24h
Flucytosine Ancobon®	250, 500 mg cap	PO	50–150 mg/kg/day	q6h
Foscarnet sodium Foscavir®	6, 12 g vials	IV	Initial: 180 mg/kg/day Maintenance: 90 mg/kg/ day	q8h q24h

Generic and Trade® Names	Dosage Form	Route	Dosage	Interval
Furazolidone Furoxone®	100 mg tab 50 mg/15 ml susp	PO	5–8 mg/kg/day	q6h
Ganciclovir sodium Cytovene®	500 mg vial 250 mg cap	IV PO	Induction: 10 mg/kg/day	q12h (1–2 hr infusion)
			Maintenance: 5 mg/kg/day (No established dosage for children)	q24h
Gentamicin sulfate Garamycin®, generic	20, 80 mg vials	IM, IV	3–7.5 mg/kg/day (cystic fibrosis 7–10); (See page 2 re q24h dosing)	q8h
Griseofulvin Fulvicin-P/G®, Grifulvin V®, Grisactin®, Gris-PEG®	Microsize: 250, 500 mg tab 125 mg/5 ml susp	PO	15 mg/kg/day	q24h
	Ultramicrosize: 125, 165, 250, 330 mg tab		6-7 mg/kg/day	q12-24h
Imipenem-Cilastatin sodium Primaxin®	250/250, 500/500 mg vials	IM, IV	40–60 mg/kg/day (Not approved for children)	q6h
Iodoquinol Yodoxin®	210, 650 mg tab	PO	40 mg/kg/day	q8h
Isoniazid Nydrazid®, generic	100, 300 mg scored tab 1 g vial 50 mg/5 ml syrup	PO, IM	10–20 mg/kg/day (max 300 mg)	q12–24h

Itraconazole Sporanox®	100 mg cap 10 mg/ml sol'n	PO	200–400 mg/day (adult dosage) ? 5 mg/kg/day	q24h
Ivermectin Stromectal®	6 mg scored tab	PO	150-200 mcg/kg	1 dose
Kanamycin sulfate	75 mg, 0.5, 1 g vials	IM, IV	15–30 mg/kg/day (See page 2 re q24h dosing)	q8h
Kantrex®, generic	500 mg cap	PO	150–250 mg/kg/day (for suppression of bowel flora)	q1–6h
Ketoconazole Nizoral®	200 mg scored tab	PO	3.3-6.6 mg/kg/day (max 800 mg/day)	q24h
Lamivudine Epivir®	150 mg tab 50 mg/5 ml sol'n	PO	8 mg/kg/day	q12h
Levofloxacin Levaquin®	250, 500 mg tab 500 mg vial	PO IV	500 mg/day (adults; not approved < 18 yrs)	q24h
Lomefloxacin HCl Maxaquin®	400 mg tab	PO	400 mg/day (adult dosage)	q24h

Generic and Trade® Names	Dosage Form	Route	Dosage	Interval
Loracarbef Lorabid®	200, 400 mg cap 100, 200 mg/5 ml susp	PO	30 (otitis)–15 (other indications) mg/kg/day	q12h
Mebendazole Vermox®	100 mg chewable tab	PO	See Section VII	
Mefloquine HCl Lariam®	250 mg scored tab	PO	See Section VII	
Meropenem Merrem®	0.5, 1g vial	IV	60 mg/kg/day (meningitis 120)	q8h
Methenamine hippurate Urex®	1 g tab	PO	25–50 mg/kg/day	q12h
Methenamine mandelate Uroquid®, generic	500 mg tab 500 mg/5 ml susp	PO	50–75 mg/kg/day	q6h
Metronidazole Flagyl®, Metric 21®, Protostat®, generic	250, 500 mg tab	PO	15–35 mg/kg/day	q8h
	500 mg vial	IV	30 mg/kg/day	q6h
Mezlocillin sodium Mezlin®	1, 2, 3, 4 g vials	IV	200–300 mg/kg/day	q4–6h
Miconazole Monistat®	200 mg amp	IV	20–40 mg/kg/day	q8h

Minocycline HCl Dynacin®, Minocin®, generic	50, 100 mg pellet-filled cap 50 mg/5 ml susp	PO	4 mg/kg/day (Pts > 7 yrs)	q12h
	100 mg vial	IV	4 mg/kg/day (Pts > 7 yrs)	q12h
Mupirocin Bactroban®, Bactroban Nasal	15, 30 g tube 1 g tube (nasal)	Topical	Apply to infected skin or nasal mucosa	q8h
Nafcillin sodium Unipen®	250 mg cap, 500 mg tab 250 mg/5 ml sol'n	PO	50–100 mg/kg/day	q6h
	0.5, 1, 2 g vials	IM, IV	150 mg/kg/day	q6h
Nalidixic acid NegGram®	0.25, 0.5, 1 g tab 250 mg/5 ml susp	PO	55 mg/kg/day	q6h
Neomycin sulfate	500 mg tab 125 mg/5 ml sol'n	PO	50–100 mg/kg/day	q6–8h
Netilmicin sulfate Netromycin®	150 mg vial	IV, IM	3–7.5 mg/kg/day (See page 2 re q24h dosing)	q8h
Niclosamide Niclocide®	500 mg chewable tab	PO	40 mg/kg/day	q24h

Generic and Trade® Names	Dosage Forms	Route	Dosage	Interval
Nitrofurantoin Furadantin®	25 mg/5 ml susp	PO	5–7 mg/kg/day	q6h
Nitrofurantoin Macrodantin®, generic	25, 50, 100 mg cap	PO	5–7 mg/kg/day	q6h
Norfloxacin Noroxin®	400 mg tab	PO	800 mg/day (adult dosage)	q12h
Nystatin Mycostatin®, generic	100,000 u/ml susp 500,000 u tab	PO (not swallowed)	Infants 2 ml/dose; Children 4–6 ml or 1 tab/dose	q6h
Ofloxacin Floxin®	200, 300, 400 mg tab 400 mg vial	PO	400–800 mg/day (adult dosage)	q12h
Oxacillin, sodium Bactocill®, Prostaphlin®, generic	250, 500 mg cap 250 mg/5 ml sol'n	PO	50–100 mg/kg/day	q6h
	0.25, 0.5, 1, 2, 4 g vials	IM, IV	150–200 mg/kg/day	q6h
Oxytetracycline HCl Terramycin®	500 mg vial with 2% lidocaine	IM	15–25 mg/kg/day	q8–12h
Paromomycin sulfate Humatin®	250 mg cap	PO	30 mg/kg/day	q8h
Penicillin G, benzathine Bicillin®	3 million unit 10 ml vial; 1, 1.5 and 2 ml syringes containing 600,000 u/ml	IM	50,000 u/kg	1 dose

Penicillin G, potassium Pfizerpen®	1, 2, 10, 20 million unit vials	IV	100,000–250,000 u/kg/day	q4h
Penicillin G, procaine Wycillin®	0.3, 0.6, 1.2. 2.4 million unit vial	IM	25,000–50,000 u/kg/day	q12–24h
	5 million unit vial	IM, IV	100,000–250,000 u/kg/day	q4h
Penicillin V Ledercillin VK®, Pen-Vee K®, V-Cillin K®, Veetids®, generic	125, 250, 500 mg tab 125, 250 mg/5 ml sol'n 125, 250 mg/5 ml drops	PO	25–50 mg/kg/day	q6–8h
Pentamidine isethionate NebuPent®, Pentam 300®	300 mg vial	IV	4 mg/kg/day	q24h
Piperacillin sodium Pipracil®	2, 3, 4 g vials	IV	200–300 mg/kg/day (Not approved for children)	q4–6h
Piperacillin/Tazobactam Zosyn®	2/.25, /.375, 4/.5 g vials	IV	240 mg PIP/kg/day (Not approved for children)	q8h
Polymyxin B sulfate Aerosporin®	50 mg (500,000 unit) vial	IM, IV	3–4.5 mg/kg/day	q6h (IM); continuous infusion (IV)

Generic and Trade® Names	Dosage Forms	Route	Dosage	Interval
Praziquantel Biltricide®	600 mg 3–scored tab	PO	50–75 mg/kg/day	q8h
Pyrantel pamoate Antiminth®	250 mg/5 ml susp	PO	11 mg/kg	1 dose
Pyrazinamide	500 mg tab	PO	30 mg/kg/day	q12–24h
Pyrimethamine (See sulfadoxine) Daraprim®	25 mg scored tab	PO	0.5–1 mg/kg/day	q12h
Quinacrine HCl (Not available in the U.S.)	100 mg cap	PO	6 mg/kg/day	q8h
Ribavirin Virazole®	6 g vial	Inhalation	1 vial by SPAG-2 aerosol generator	q24h
Rifabutin Mycobutin®	150 mg cap	PO	300 mg/day (adult dosage)	q12–24h
Rifampin Rifadin®, Rimactane®	150, 300 mg cap 600 mg vial	PO IV	10–20 mg/kg/day (max 600 mg)	q12–24h
Rimantadine HCl Flumadine®	100 mg tab 50 mg/5 ml syrup	PO	5 mg/kg/day (max 150 mg/day)	q24h
Ritonavir Norvir®	100 mg cap 80 mg/ml oral sol'n	PO	1200 mg/day (adult dosage)	q12h

Saquinavir mesylate Invirase®	200 mg cap	PO	1800 mg/day (adult dosage)	q8h
Sparfloxacin Zagan®	200 mg tab	PO	400 mg 1st dose; then 200 mg/day (adult dosage; not approved for < 18 yrs)	q24h
Spectinomycin HCl Trobicin®	2, 4 g vials	IM	30–40 mg/kg	1 dose
Stavudine (d4T) Zerit®	15, 20, 30, 40 mg cap 5 mg/5 ml sol'n	PO	0.125–4 mg/kg/day	q12–24h
Streptomycin sulfate	1 g vials	IM	20–30 mg/kg/day	q12h
Sulfadiazine	0.3, 0.5 g tab	PO	120–150 mg/kg/day	q4–6h
Sulfadoxine and pyrimethamine Fansidar®	500 mg SDX + 25 mg PMA scored tab	PO	See Section VII	
Sulfamethizole Thiosulfil Forte®	0.5 g tab	PO	30–45 mg/kg/day	q6h
Sulfamethoxazole Gantanol®, generic	0.5 g tab 0.5 g/5 ml susp	PO	50–60 mg/kg/day	q12h

Generic and Trade® Names	Dosage Form	Route	Dosage	Interval
Sulfasalazine Azulfidine®, generic	500 mg tab	PO	30–60 mg/kg/day	q4–8h
Sulfisoxazole Gantrisin®, generic	0.5 g tab 0.5 g/5 ml susp or syrup	PO	120–150 mg/kg/day	q4–6h
Tetracycline Achromycin®, Sumycin®, generic	250, 500 mg cap, tab 125 mg/5 ml syrup 125, 250 mg/5 ml susp	PO	25–50 mg/kg/day (pts > 7 yrs)	q6h
Thiabendazole Mintezol®	500 mg chewable, scored tab 500 mg/5 ml susp	PO	50 mg/kg/day	q12h
Ticarcillin disodium Ticar®	1, 3, 6 g vials	IV	200–300 mg/kg/day	q4–6h
Ticarcillin and clavulanate potassium Timentin®	3/0.1, 3/0.2 g vials	IV	200–300 mg/kg/day (Not approved for children)	q4–6h
Tobramycin sulfate Nebcin®, generic	20, 80 mg, 1.2 g vials	IV, IM	3–7.5 mg/kg/day (cystic fibrosis 7–10) (See page 2 re q24h dosing)	q8h
Trifluridine Viroptic®	1% ophthal sol'n	Topical	1 drop (max 9 drops/day)	q2h
Trimethoprim Proloprim®, generic	100 mg scored tab	PO	4-10 mg/kg/day (Not approved for children)	q12h

Trimethoprim-Sulfamethoxazole Bactrim®, Cotrim®, Septra®, Sulfatrim®, generic	80 mg TMP/400 mg SMX tab 160 mg TMP/800 mg SMX tab 40 mg TMP/200 mg SMX/5 ml susp	PO	8–12 mg TMP/ 40–60 mg SMX/kg/day; (20 mg TMP/100 mg SMX/kg/day for *Pneumocystis)*	q12h q6h
	400 mg TMP/2000 mg SMX amp	IV		
Trimetrexate glucuronate Neutrexin®	25 mg/5 ml vial	IV	45 mg/m^2 (adult dose); <u>Must</u> be given with leukovorin	q24h
Troleandomycin Tao®	250 mg cap	PO	25–40 mg/kg/day	q6h
Valacyclovir HCl Valtrex®	500 mg cap	PO	Herpes simplex: 1000 mg/day Herpes zoster: 3000 mg/day (adult dosage)	q12h
Vancomycin HCl Vancocin®, generic	1, 10 g bottle 125, 250 mg cap	PO	10–50 mg/kg/day (Oral use not recommended)	q6h
	0.5, 1 g vials	IV	40 mg/kg/day (meningitis 60) as 1 hr infusion	q6h

Generic and Trade® Names	Dosage Form	Route	Dosage	Interval
Vidarabine Vira-A®	3% ophthalmic ointment	Topical	Approx 1 cm of ointment	q3h
	1 g vial	IV	10–30 mg/kg/day	q24h
Zalcitabine (ddC) HIVID®	0.375, 0.750 mg tab	PO	2.25 mg/day (adult dosage)	q8h
Zidovudine (AZT) Retrovir®	200 mg vial 100 mg cap 50 mg/5 ml syrup	IV PO	720 mg/m^2/day (max 800 mg/day)	q6h

IX. ALPHABETICAL LISTING OF TRADE NAMES

Trade Name (Drug Company)
--Generic Name

- A -

ABELCET (Liposome Co.)
--Amphotericin B, lipsomal
Achromycin (Wyeth-Lederle)
--Tetracycline
Aerosporin (Glaxo Wellcome)
--Polymyxin B
Albenza (SmithKline Beecham)
--Albendazole
Amoxil (SmithKline Beecham)
--Amoxicillin
AMPHOTEC (Gensia)
--amphotericin B cholesteryl sulfate
Ancef (SmithKline Beecham)
--Cefazolin
Ancobon (Roche)
--Flucytosine
Antiminth (Pfizer)
--Pyrantel pamoate
Aralen (Sanofi Winthrop)
--Cloroquine
Aralen with Primaquine (Sanofi Winthrop)
--Cloroquine/primaquine
A/T/S (Hoechst Marion Roussel)
--2% erythromycin sol'n (Topical)
Augmentin (SmithKline Beecham)
--Amoxicillin/clavulanate potassium
Aureomycin (Wyeth-Lederle)
--Chlortetracycline (Topical)
Azactam (Bristol-Myers Squibb)
--Aztreonam
Azo Gantanol (Roche)
--Sulfamethoxazole/phenazopyridine
Azo Gantrisin (Roche)
--Sulfisoxazole/phenazopyridine
Azulfidine (Pharmacia and Upjohn)
--Sulfasalazine

- B -

Bactocill (SmithKline Beecham)
--Oxacillin
Bactrim (Roche)
--Trimethoprim/sulfamethoxazole
Bactroban (SmithKline Beecham)
--Mupirocin (Topical)
Benemid (Merck)
--Probenecid
Biaxin (Abbott)
--Clarithromycin
Bicillin (Wyeth-Lederle)
--Benzathine penicillin G
Biltricide (Bayer)
--Praziquantel
Biocef (Interferon Sciences)
--Cephalexin

- C -

Ceclor (Lilly)
--Cefaclor
Cedax (Schering)
--Ceftibuten
Cefizox (Fujisawa)
--Ceftizoxime
Cefobid (Roerig)
--Cefoperazone
Cefotan (Zeneca)
--Cefotetan
Ceftin (Glaxo Wellcome)
--Cefuroxime axetil
Cefzil (BristolMyers Squibb)
--Cefprozil
Ceptaz (Glaxo Wellcome)
--Ceftazidime
Chibroxin (Merck)
--Norfloxacin ophthalmalic sol'n
Chloromycetin (Parke-Davis)
--Chloramphenicol

Cinobac (Oclassen)
--Cinoxacin
Cipro (Bayer)
--Ciprofloxacin
Claforan (Hoechst Marion Roussel)
--Cefotaxime
Cleocin (Pharmacia and Upjohn)
--Clindamycin
Coly-Mycin (Parke-Davis)
--Colistin
Cotrim (Teva)
--Trimethoprim/sulfamethoxazole
Cytovene (Syntex)
--Ganciclovir

- D -

Dapsone USP (Jacobus)
--Dapsone
Daraprim (Glaxo Wellcome)
--Pyrimethamine
Declomycin (Wyeth-Lederle)
--Demeclocycline
Denavir (SmithKline Beecham)
--Penciclovir 1% cream
Diflucan (Roerig)
--Fluconazole
Doryx (Parke-Davis)
--Doxycycline
Duricef (Bristol-Myers Squibb)
--Cefadroxil
Dycill (SmithKline Beecham)
--Dicloxacillin
Dynabac (Lilly)
--Dirithromycin
DYNACIN (Medicis)
--Minocycline

- E -

E. E. S. (Abbott)
--Erythromycin ethylsuccinate
Elimite Cream (Allergan Herbert)
--Permethrin 5% (Topical)
E-Mycin (Boots)
--Erythromycin
Epivir (Glaxo Wellcome)
--Lamivudine
ERYC (Parke-Davis)
--Erythromycin
Erygel (Allergan Herbert)
--2% erythromycin gel (Topical)
EryPed (Abbott)
--Erythromycin ethylsuccinate
Ery-Tab (Abbott)
--Erythromycin
Erythrocin (Abbott)
--Erythromycin stearate
Eryzole (Alra)
--Erythromycin ethylsuccinate/ sulfisoxazole acetyl

- F -

Famvir (SmithKline Beecham)
--Famciclovir
Fansidar (Roche)
--Sulfadoxine/pyrimethamine
Flagyl (Searle)
--Metronidazole
Floxin (McNeil)
--Ofloxacin
Flumadine (Forest)
--Rimantadine
Fortaz (Glaxo Wellcome)
--Ceftazidime
Foscavir (Astra)
--Foscarnet
Fulvicin (Schering)
--Griseofulvin
Fungizone (Apothecon)
--Amphotericin B
Furacin (Roberts)
--Nitrofurazone (Topical)
Furadantin (Procter & Gamble)
--Nitrofurantoin
Furoxone (Roberts)
--Furazolidone

- G -

Gantanol (Roche)
--Sulfamethoxazole
Gantrisin (Roche)
--Sulfisoxazole

Garamycin (Schering)
--Gentamicin
Geocillin (Roerig)
--Carbenicillin indanyl
Grifulvin V (Ortho)
--Griseofulvin
Grisactin (Wyeth-Lederle)
--Griseofulvin
Gris-PEG (Allergan Herbert)
--Griseofulvin

- H -

HIVID (Roche)
--Zalcitabine
Humatin (Parke-Davis)
--Paromomycin

- I -

Ilosone (Dista)
--Erythromycin estolate
Ilotycin (Dista)
--Erythromycin
Ilotycin Gluceptate (Dista)
--Erythromycin gluceptate
Invirase (Roche)
--Saquinavir

- K -

Kantrex (Apothecon)
--Kanamycin
Keflex (Dista)
--Cephalexin
Keflin (Lilly)
--Cephalothin
Keftab (Dista)
--Cephalexin
Kefurox (Lilly)
--Cefuroxime
Kefzol (Lilly)
--Cefazolin

- L -

Lamprene (Geigy)
--Clofazimine
Lariam (Roche)
--Mefloquine
Ledercillin (Wyeth-Lederle)
--Penicillin VK
Levaquin (Ortho-McNeil)
--Levofloxacin
Lorabid (Lilly)
--Loracarbef
Lotrimin (Schering)
--Clotrimazole (Topical)

- M -

Macrodantin (Procter & Gamble)
--Nitrofurantoin
Mandol (Lilly)
--Cefamandole
Maxaquin (Searle)
--Lomefloxacin
Maxipime (BristolMyers Squibb)
--Cefipime
Mefoxin (Merck)
--Cefoxitin
Mepron (Glaxo Wellcome)
--Atovaquone
Merrem (Zeneca)
--Meropenem
Metric-21 (Fielding)
--Metronidazole
Mezlin (Bayer)
--Mezlocillin
Minocin (Wyeth-Lederle)
--Minocycline
Mintezol (Merck)
--Thiabendazole
Monistat (Ortho; Janssen)
--Miconazole
Monocid (SmithKline Beecham)
--Cefonicid
Myambutol (Wyeth-Lederle)
--Ethambutol
Mycelex (Bayer)
--Clotrimazole
Mycobutin (Pharmacia and Upjohn)
--Rifabutin
Mycostatin (BristolMyers Squibb)
--Nystatin

- N -

Nebcin (Lilly)
--Tobramycin
NebuPent (Fujisawa)
--Pentamidine aerosol
NegGram (Sanofi Winthrop)
--Nalidixic acid
Neosporin (Glaxo Wellcome)
--Neomycin, polymyxin B (Topical)
Netromycin (Schering)
--Netilmicin
Neutrexin (US Bioscience)
--Trimetrexate
Niclocide (Bayer)
--Niclosamide
Nix Creme Rinse (Glaxo Wellcome)
--Permethrim 1% (Topical)
Nizoral (Janssen)
--Ketoconazole
Noroxin (Merck)
--Norfloxacin
Norvir (Abbott)
--Ritonavir
Nydrazid (Apothecon)
--Isoniazid

- O -

Omnipen (Wyeth-Lederle)
--Ampicillin

- P -

PCE Dispertab (Abbott)
--Erythromycin particles in tablets
Pediazole (Ross)
--Erythromycin ethylsuccinate/
sulfisoxazole acetyl
Penetrex (Rhone-Poulenc Rorer)
--Enoxacin
Pentacef (SmithKline Beecham)
--Ceftazidime
Pentam 300 (Fujisawa)
--Pentamidine isethionate
Pen-Vee K (Wyeth-Lederle)
--Penicillin V
Pfizerpen (Roerig)
--Penicillin G
Pipracil (Wyeth-Lederle)
--Piperacillin
Plaquenil (Sanofi Winthrop)
--Hydroxychloroquine
Polysporin (Glaxo Wellcome)
--Polymyxin B/bacitracin (Topical)
Polytrim Ophthalmic Solution (Allergan)
--Trimethoprim and polymyxin B
(Topical)
Primaxin (Merck)
--Imipenem-cilastatin
Proloprim (Glaxo Wellcome)
--Trimethoprim
Prostaphlin (Apothecon)
--Oxacillin
Protostat (Ortho)
--Metronidazole
Pyrazinamide (Wyeth-Lederle)
--Pyrazinamide

- R -

Retrovir (Glaxo Wellcome)
--Zidovudine
Rifadin (Hoechst Marion Roussel)
--Rifampin
Rifamate (Hoechst Marion Roussel)
--Rifampin/isoniazid
Rimactane (Ciba)
--Rifampin
Rocephin (Roche)
--Ceftriaxone

- S -

Septra (Glaxo Wellcome)
--Trimethoprim/sulfamethoxazole
Seromycin (Lilly)
--Cycloserine
Sodium Sulamyd (Schering)
--Sodium sulfacetamide (Topical)
Spectrobid (Roerig)
--Bacampicillin

Sporanox (Janssen)
--Itraconazole
Stromectal (Merck)
--Ivermectin
Sulfatrim (Barre-National)
--Trimethoprim-sulfamethoxazole
Sumycin (Apothecon)
--Tetracycline
Suprax (Wyeth-Lederle)
--Cefixime
Symmetrel (DuPont)
--Amantadine

- T -

Tao (Roerig)
--Troleandomycin
Tazicef (SmithKline Beecham)
--Ceftazidime
Tazidime (Lilly)
--Ceftazidime
Terramycin (Roerig)
--Oxytetracycline
Thiosulfil Forte (Wyeth-Lederle)
--Sulfamethizole
Ticar (SmithKline Beecham)
--Ticarcillin
Tice BCG Vaccine (Organon)
--BCG Vaccine
Timentin (SmithKline Beecham)
--Ticarcillin/clavulanate
Topicycline (Roberts)
--Tetracycline (Topical)
Trecator-SC (Wyeth-Lederle)
--Ethionamide
Trobicin (Pharmacia and Upjohn)
--Spectinomycin

- U -

Unasyn (Roerig)
--Ampicillin/sulbactam
Unipen (Wyeth-Lederle)
--Nafcillin
Urex (3M)
--Methenamine hipprate
Urobiotic (Roerig)
--Oxytetracycline, sulfamethizole/ phenazopyridine
Uroquid-Acid (Beach)
--Methenamine/sodium acid phosphate

- V -

Valtrex (Glaxo Wellcome)
--Valacyclovir
Vancocin (Lilly)
--Vancomycin
Vantin (Pharmacia and Upjohn)
--Cefpodoxime proxetil
V-Cillin K (Lilly)
--Penicillin V
Veetids (Apothecon)
--Penicillin V
Vermox (Janssen)
--Mebendazole
Vibramycin (Roerig, Pfizer)
--Doxycycline
Vibra-Tabs (Pfizer)
--Doxycycline
Videx (BristolMyers Squibb)
--Didanosine
Vira-A (Parke-Davis)
--Vidarabine
Virazole (ICN)
--Ribavirin
Viroptic (Glaxo Wellcome)
--Trifluridine (Ophthalmic)

- W -

Wycillin (Wyeth-Lederle)
--Penicillin G procaine
Wymox (Wyeth-Lederle)
--Amoxicillin

- Y -

Yodoxin (Glenwood)
--Iodoquinol (formerly diiodohydroxyquin)

- Z -

Zagam (Rhône-Poulenc Rorer)
--Sparfloxacin
Zefazone (Pharmacia and Upjohn)
--Cefmetazole
Zerit (BristolMyers Squibb)
--Stavudine
Zinacef (Glaxo Wellcome)
--Cefuroxime
Zithromax (Pfizer)
--Azithromycin
Zosyn (Wyeth-Lederle)
--Piperacillin/tazobactam
Zovirax (Glaxo Wellcome)
--Acyclovir

X. PENICILLIN DESENSITIZATION

Studies have shown that an oral regimen is safer and more effective than graduated injections for desensitization to penicillins. (Pediatr Infect Dis 1982;1:344)

Penicillin V suspension is used. Signed, informed consent is recommended. An intravenous catheter is in place and emergency resuscitation materials at hand for the unlikely event of anaphylaxis. Medical personnel capable of managing anaphylaxis should be available. Doses are given at 15 minute intervals; the total regimen requires 4 hours.

Doses	Penicillin V units/ml	Amount q15 min
1–7	1,000	Doubling doses from 0.1 ml (100 units) to 6.4 ml (6,400 units)
8–10	10,000	Doubling doses from 1.2 ml (12,000 units) to 4.8 ml (48,000 units)
11–14	80,000	Doubling doses from 1.0 ml (80,000 units) to 8.0 ml (640,000 units)

(Source: N Engl J Med 1985;312:1229)

Minor allergic reactions are suppressed with epinephrine or antihistamines. Therapy is not interrupted unless there is a severe or unsuppressible reaction. If there are interruptions in therapy of more than 8 hours, it is advisable to repeat the desensitization regimen.

If the patient cannot tolerate oral medication, parenteral desensitization can be used. The method is reviewed in J Allergy Clin Immunol 1982;69:275.

XI. SEQUENTIAL PARENTERAL-ORAL ANTIBIOTIC THERAPY FOR SERIOUS INFECTIONS

Bacterial pneumonias, endocarditis and bone and joint infections often require prolonged antibiotic therapy. Intravenous therapy is unpleasant for the child and carries a hazard of nosocomial infection.

Rationale:

1. Comparable dosages of analogous parenteral and oral medications result in comparable serum concentrations from 1 to 6 hours after a dose and comparable bioavailability ("area-under-the-curve") in most patients.
2. There is no known therapeutic advantage to the momentary high serum concentrations that occur during IV administration.
3. Although the protein binding of many oral formulations is greater than that of parenteral formulations, this does not prevent good penetration into body fluid compartments.

Method:

1. Initial parenteral therapy is as follows:
   a. Alert laboratory to save pathogen for serum bactericidal tests.
   b. Perform any necessary surgical procedures.
2. Subsequent oral therapy when clinical condition is stable and patient can take and retain oral medication (usually 5-7 days) is as follows:
   a. Select appropriate oral antibiotic based on *in vitro* susceptibilities and compliance factors (mainly palatability of suspension formulations).
   b. BEGIN WITH DOSAGE 2–3 TIMES "NORMAL" DOSAGE: e.g. 75–100 MG/KG/DAY OF DICLOXACILLIN AND 100–150 MG/ KG/DAY OF OTHER BETA-LACTAMS.
   c. Serum for bactericidal titer or measurement of antibiotic concentration 1-2 hours after a dose.

NOTES:

1. The serum bactericidal titer is done quantitatively and is defined as $\geq$ 99.9% killing. For staphylococcal infections the serum bactericidal titer should be at least 1:8. For highly susceptible bacteria, such as pneumococci and Group A streptococci, titers are usually greater than 1:32. Peak serum antibiotic concentration should be $\geq$ 20 μg/ml for beta-lactams and $\geq$ 10 μg/ml for clindamycin. (NOTE: Measuring bactericidal titers is labor-intensive and difficult to standardize. Measuring antibiotic is usually pereferable.)
2. Peak serum activity usually is found 45–60 minutes after a dose taken as suspension and 1–2 hours after a capsule or tablet.
3. Approximately 5–10% of patients are unsuitable for this regimen because of poor gastrointestinal absorption of antibiotics.

WARNING: ORAL THERAPY REGIMENS FOR SERIOUS INFECTIONS ARE POTENTIALLY HAZARDOUS UNLESS ADEQUACY OF SERUM BACTERICIDAL ACTIVITY OR ANTIBIOTIC CONTENT IS MONITORED.

XII. ANTIBIOTIC THERAPY IN PATIENTS WITH RENAL FAILURE

Most antimicrobials are excreted primarily by the kidneys; therefore, when significant renal functional impairment is present, either downward adjustments in dosages must be made or the intervals between doses must be lengthened. Exceptions are drugs such as chloramphenicol that are metabolized to antibiotically inactive conjugates and those excreted primarily by the liver, such as nafcillin and ceftriaxone.

Degrees of dosage adjustment necessary for treating patients with renal failure are as follows: Major adjustments in dosage and dosing intervals are necessary for treating renal failure patients with aminoglycosides, flucytosine, and vancomycin. No adjustments in dosage are necessary in the use of amphotericin B, cefoperazone, chloramphenicol, cloxacillin, dicloxacillin, doxycyline, erythromycin, isoniazid, metronidazole, minocycline, nafcillin, and rifampin. For other antibiotics minor to moderate adjustments are necessary.

The most satisfactory way to use drugs in children with decreased renal function is by monitoring the antibiotic concentrations in serum. The customary initial loading dose is given. Initially, until antibiotic assay results are available, one makes estimates of appropriate dosage based on past experience of rates of excretion related to the degree of renal failure. Three or four serum specimens are collected at intervals over a 12–24 hour period for assay of antibiotic content. The serum half-life is estimated. The interval of dosing is every three half-lives for patients with moderate renal dysfunction and every two half-lives for those with severe renal failure; subsequent dosages are two-thirds or one-half, respectively, of the initial loading dose.

CLINICAL PHARMACISTS HAVE COMPUTER PROGRAMS FOR ANTIBIOTIC DOSAGE MODIFICATION BASED ON CREATINE CLEARANCE OR SERUM CREATINE.

Patients undergoing dialysis need additional doses after the procedure if a substantial amount of drug is removed by dialysis. With peritoneal dialysis < 10% of drug is removed in the case of most antibiotics. The exceptions are aminoglycosides (20–25%), cefazolin and cefuroxime (20%), and moxalactam and vancomycin (15–20%).

Removed by Hemodialysis	Beta-lactams	Other Drugs
> 50%	Many cephalosporins (see exceptions below), imipenem	Acyclovir, aminoglycosides, flucytosine, isoniazid, spectinomycin sulfonamides, trimethoprim
20–50%	Most penicillins (see exceptions below), aztreonam, cefaclor, ceforanide, cefapirin, moxalactam	Ethambutol, metronidazole, vancomycin
< 10%	Cefixime, cefonicid, cefoperazone, cefotetan, cloxacillin, dicloxacillin, methicillin, nafcillin, oxacillin	Amphotericin B, fluoroquinolones, macrolides, miconazole, polymyxins, tetracyclines

XIII. DILUTIONS OF ANTIBIOTICS FOR INTRAVENOUS USE

Notes: 1. Manufacturers' recommendations for dilution of antibiotics for intravenous use sometimes are not appropriate for pediatric patients because of volumes of fluid that are unsuitably large for the desired time of infusion. The dilutions given below should result in convenient volumes, and they are well-tolerated in terms of not causing irritation of veins. These recommendations were prepared by the clinical pharmacists at Children's Medical Center, Dallas.

2. Check the manufacturer's instructions for compatible IV solutions.

	Concentration in mg/ml for:		
Antibiotics	**Central Catheter**	**Peripheral vein**	**Duration of Infusion (minutes)**
Beta-lactams			
Ampicillin, mezlocillin, ticarcillin, ceftriaxone, cefuroxime	100	50	15–30
Cefepime	40	40	30
Meropenem	50	50	15–30
Nafcillin	100	40	15–30
Imipenem	5	5	30–60
Pencillin G	1 mil units/ml	50,000 units/ml	15–30
Aminoglycosides			
Amikacin	5	5	30
Gentamicin, tobramycin	40	40	30
Kanamycin	6	5	30
Others			
Acyclovir	10	7	60–180
Amphotericin B	0.25	0.1	120–240
Aztreonam	66	20	> 6 mg/kg/min
Chloramphenicol	100	50	30
Ciprofloxacin	2	2	60
Clindamycin	18	18	15–30
Fluconazole	2	2	≤ 3 mg/min
Foscarnet	24	12	60
Ganciclovir	10	10	60
Metronidazole	6	6	30–60
Trimethoprim	1.6	1	60
Rifampin	6	3	≥ 60
Vancomycin	5	5	60–120
Zidovudine	4	4	60

XIV. MAXIMUM DOSAGES FOR LARGE CHILDREN

Infants and young children have a large volume of distribution of many antibiotics in the body. This means that, in order to achieve good serum concentrations, we give larger doses based on body weight or surface area than are given to adults. The following dosages of commonly used drugs should not be exceeded except in special circumstances. (See p 97 for oral therapy of serious infections.)

Maximum Daily Dosage	Antimicrobials
ORAL FORMULATIONS	
4–8 g	Sulfisoxazole
2–3 g	Amoxicillin, ampicillin, carbenicillin, cephalexin, cephradine, cloxacillin, cyclacillin, lincomycin, nafcillin, oxacillin, penicillin G or V, tetracycline
1–2 g	Cefaclor, cefprozil, cefuroxime axetil, ciprofloxacin, clindamycin, dicloxacillin, erythromycin, metronidazole
0.5–1.2 g	Loracarbef, trimethoprim
400 mg	Cefixime, cefpodoxime
PARENTERAL FORMULATIONS	
30–40 g	Carbenicillin
18–24 g	Azlocillin, mezlocillin, piperacillin, ticarcillin
10–12 g	Ampicillin, cefotaxime, ceftizoxime, cephalothin, methicillin, moxalactam, nafcillin, oxacillin
6–8 g	Aztreonam, ceftazidime
4–6 g	Cefamandole, cefoperazone, cefazolin, cefuroxime, meropenem
2–4 g	Cefepime, ceftriaxone, chloramphenicol, clindamycin, erythromycin, metronidazole, spectinomycin, vancomycin
1–2 g	Amikacin, cefonicid, ceforanide, streptomycin
0.75–1 g	Kanamycin, lincomycin
500 mg	Gentamicin, netilmicin, tobramycin
20 million units	Penicillin G
4.8 million units	Penicillin G, procaine
2.4 million units	Penicillin G, benzathine

XV. DOSAGES BASED ON BODY SURFACE AREA

Antibiotic dosages calculated on the basis of body weight are not always appropriate for obese and malnourished patients. (Obese patients would have excessively high serum concentrations, and malnourished patients would have lower than desired serum concentrations.) For such patients dosages calculated from body surface area are preferred.

Calculation of body surface area (J Pediatr 1978;93:62)

B.S.A. (m^2) = wt (kg)$^{0.5378}$ x ht (cm)$^{0.3964}$ x 0.024265, which can be solved using logarithms on a pocket calculator as:

$$\log \text{B.S.A.} = \log \text{wt} \times 0.5378 + \log \text{ht} \times 0.3964 + \log 0.024265$$

Antibiotics (IM or IV)	Each Dose/m^2	Interval	Amt/m^2/24 hrs
Aminoglycoside			
Amikacin, kanamycin	200 mg	q8h	600 mg
gentamicin, netilmicin, tobramycin	60 mg	q8h	180 mg
Beta-Lactams			
Penicillin G (meningitis)	1,750,000 u	q4h	10,500,000 u
Penicillin G (others)	450,000 u	q4h	2,700,000 u
Ampicillin, methicillin, oxacillin, cephalothin	1.4 g	q6h	5.6 g
Ceftriaxone	1.4 g	q12h	2.8 g
Ceftazidime, moxalactam	1.4 g	q8h	4.2 g
Nafcillin, cefamandole, cefotaxime, ceftizoxime	1.05 g	q6h	4.2 g
Cefazolin, cefuroxime	0.8 g	q8h	2.4 g
Cefonicid, ceforanide	0.55 g	q12h	1.1 g
Carbenicillin	4 g	q6h	16 g
Ticarcillin, azlocillin, mezlocillin, piperacillin	2.5 g	q6h	10 g
Aztreonam	0.8 g	q6h	3.2 g
Imipenem	0.55 g	q6h	2.2 g
Miscellaneous			
Chloramphenicol (meningitis)	0.7 g	q6h	2.8 g
Chloramphenicol (others)	0.45 g	q6h	1.8 g
Metronidazole	280 mg	q8h	840 mg
Sulfamethoxazole	0.5 g	q8h	1.5 g
Trimethoprim	100 mg	q8h	300 mg
Vancomycin (CNS infection)	0.425 g	q6h	1.7 g
Vancomycin (others)	0.275 g	q6h	1.1 g
Zidovudine	160 mg	q6h	640 mg

XVI. ADVERSE REACTIONS TO ANTIMICROBIAL AGENTS

A good rule of clinical practice is to be suspicious of an adverse drug reaction when a patient's clinical course deviates from the expected. This section focuses on reactions that require close observation or laboratory monitoring either because of their frequency or because of their severity. For detailed listings of reactions, consult the package inserts.

Beta-Lactam Antibiotics. The most feared reaction to penicillins, anaphylactic shock, is extremely rare, and no absolutely reliable means of predicting its occurrence exists. The commercially available skin testing material, benzylpenicilloylpolylysine (Pre-Pen®), should be used in conjunction with the Minor Determinant Mixture (MDM) and penicilloic acid skin testing, but the latter two are not commercially available. A dilute solution of penicillin G (10,000 u/ml) can be used as a skin test material in place of MDM. If the scratch test and intradermal test with 0.01 ml are negative, penicillin of the same lot number should be used for administration to the patient. (Be prepared to treat anaphylaxis.) If the allergic status is questionable one can use a desensitization schedule (See Section X). The monobactam, aztreonam, does not exhibit cross-sensitization with penicillins and cephalosporins.

Ampicillin and other aminopenicillins cause minor adverse effects frequently. Oral or diaper area candidiasis, diarrhea and morbilliform, and blotchy "ampicillin rashes" are common. The latter is not allergic in origin and is not a contraindication to subsequent use of ampicillin or any other penicillin. Diarrhea is somewhat less common with amoxicillin and more common with Augmentin®, but the new 7:1 formulation of Augmentin causes less diarrhea than the original formulation did. Rarely beta-lactams cause serious, life-threatening pseudomembranous enterocolitis due to suppression of normal bowel flora and overgrowth with *Clostridium difficile*. Drug fever is probably more common with ampicillin than with other penicillins. Serum sickness is uncommon. Pancytopenia is rare, and reversible neutropenia and thrombocytopenia occasionally occur with any of the beta-lactams.

Nephrotoxicity is probably most common with methicillin (approximately 5%) but has been reported with all the penicillins (rarest with nafcillin). Laboratory monitoring should be performed. Hemorrhagic cystitis occurs mainly in poorly hydrated patients receiving large dosages and is probably a direct irritant effect of the large concentrations of drug in urine. It disappears even with continued use of the antibiotic when the patient's urine output increases. Ticarcillin interferes with platelet function but generally does not cause clinical bleeding problems. Hypokalemia with ticarcillin is more common than with other beta-lactams. Mezlocillin and piperacillin appear to have similar adverse effects to ticarcillin with the exception that mezlocillin has the least effect on platelet function.

Imipenem-cilastatin has similar adverse effects to other beta-lactams. In addition, patients occasionally have CNS reactions (convulsions, hallucinations, altered affect). Convulsions are most likely in the elderly or in patients with CNS disease, especially neonates. Meropenem does not have the undesirable CNS effects seen with imipenem.

The cephalosporins for oral use are generally better tolerated than the penicillins. The cephalosporins can cause a direct Coombs' reaction in the blood, but this is of no known clinical significance. Most cephalosporins are painful on IM injection and can cause phlebothrombosis with IV administration. Cefazolin and cefuroxime are better tolerated IM, and cefamandole and cephradine appear to cause fewer problems on IV use than the others. Cefaclor has been associated with a transient serum sickness-like reaction (rash, arthralgia); the cause is unknown. Similarly, a serum sickness-like reaction has been reported with IV use of cephapirin. Cefoperazone and cefamandole can cause a disulfiram (Antabuse)-like effect; patients should avoid alcohol, including elixirs. Prolonged prothrombin time and bleeding episodes have also been attributed to those drugs. It is treatable (and probably preventable) with vitamin K. The third generation cephalosporins cause profound alteration of normal flora on mucosal surfaces, and all have caused pseudomembranous colitis on rare occasions. Ceftriaxone commonly causes loose stools, but it is rarely severe enough to require stopping therapy. Ceftriaxone can cause sludging in the gallbladder (a calcium complex of ceftriaxone) which, on rare occasions, causes symptoms and jaundice; this is reversible after stopping the drug. Ceftriaxone is also reported to displace bilirubin from albumin-binding sites.

Aminoglycosides. Any of the aminoglycosidic aminocyclitol antibiotics can cause serious nephrotoxicity and ototoxicity. (The closely related aminocyclitol, spectinomycin, is safer in this respect.) The newer aminoglycosides (amikacin, tobramycin, gentamicin and netilmicin) are generally safer than kanamycin, streptomycin or neomycin. In animal studies, netilmicin is the least ototoxic. Monitor all patients receiving aminoglycoside therapy for renal toxicity with periodic urinalyses and determinations of the BUN and creatinine and be alert to ototoxicity. Common practice is to measure the serum concentration one-half to one hour after a dose to make sure one is in a safe and therapeutic range and to measure a trough serum concentration immediately preceding a dose. Monitoring is especially important in patients with any degree of renal insufficiency. Elevated trough concentrations (> 2 μg/ml for gentamicin, netilmicin and tobramycin and >10 μg/ml for amikacin and kanamycin) should be avoided. (With once daily administration regimens, peak values are 2–3 times greater.) Aminoglycosides potentiate botulinum toxin.

The "loop" diuretics (ethacrynic acid, furosemide, piretanide and bumetanide) potentiate the ototoxicity of the aminoglycosides. The "non-loop" diuretics (hydrodiuril, mercuhydrin and mannitol) do not interact with aminoglycosides to produce ototoxicity. Nephrotoxicity may be less common with once daily (as opposed to thrice daily) dosing regimens.

The aminoglycosides are well tolerated via intramuscular and intravenous routes of administration. Minor side effects such as rashes, drug fever, etc. are rare.

Chloramphenicol. The most feared toxicity of chloramphenicol, irreversible aplastic anemia, is very rare. It has been said that aplastic anemia is more likely with oral than with parenteral chloramphenicol, but documenting that claim is difficult, and it is probably incorrect. Regardless of the route of administration, laboratory monitoring for hematologic toxicity should be carried out in patients treated with chloramphenicol. Transient pharmacologic bone marrow depression occurs in almost all patients receiving large dosages (> 75 mg/kg/day) of chloramphenicol. As long as the absolute neutrophil count remains more than 1,500 per μl and the platelet count above 100,000 per μl, one can continue to administer chloramphenicol if it is necessary. These hematologic changes reverse rapidly when the drug is stopped.

The "gray syndrome" with potentially fatal circulatory collapse is due to excessive accumulation of chloramphenicol in neonates secondary to delayed conjugation (because of inadequate glucuronyl transferase activity) and poor renal excretion of unconjugated chloramphenicol. Chloramphenicol should not be used in neonates unless there are no suitable alternative drugs; dosage must be restricted and, ideally, one would monitor serum concentrations (therapeutic range 10–25 μg/ml). Phenobarbitol induces glucuronidative enzymes so that patients receiving phenobarbitol may require larger than normal doses of chloramphenicol. Rifampin has a similar effect. Concomitant phenytoin administration often causes accumulation of chloramphenicol in serum, which may reach a toxic concentration; conversely, accumulation of phenytoin to toxic concentrations has also been reported. Other drugs metabolized by the liver, such as theophylline, acetaminophen and isoniazid, could have similar effects.

Minor side effects such as nausea and diarrhea are rare. With prolonged use (principally in children with cystic fibrosis), optic neuritis and peripheral neuritis have occurred. Alteration of normal respiratory and gastrointestinal flora may lead to infection with opportunistic bacteria or fungi. Drug fever is rare.

Tetracyclines. Tetracyclines should be used infrequently in pediatric patients because the major indications are uncommon diseases (rickettsial infections, brucellosis), with the exception of acne, chlamydial infections and Lyme disease. Side effects include minor gastrointestinal disturbances, photosensitization, angioedema, browning of the tongue, glossitis, pruritis ani, and exfoliative dermatitis. The diarrhea associated with tetracycline administration may be a direct irritant effect or due to alteration of normal GI flora with overgrowth of opportunistic bacteria or fungi. Alterations in normal respiratory tract flora produced by tetracycline increase the risk of superinfections by staphylococci and other opportunistic organisms.

Toxic effects from tetracyclines involve virtually every organ system. Hepatic and pancreatic injury have occurred with accidental overdosage and in patients with renal failure. (Pregnant women are particularly at risk for hepatic injury.) Tetracyclines are deposited in growing bones and teeth with depression of linear bone growth, dental staining and defects in enamelization in deciduous and permanent teeth. This effect is dose-related and the risk extends up to 8 years of age. Patients taking outdated, degraded tetracycline can develop a Fanconi renal syndrome. Pseudotumor cerebri of unknown cause has rarely been seen in young infants who receive normal therapeutic doses. Minocycline causes dose-related vestibular toxicity in adults. Tetracycline is painful and irritative when injected into muscle, and thrombophlebitis occurs if the drug is given IV too rapidly.

Macrolides. Erythromycin is one of the safest antimicrobial agents. It commonly produces nausea and epigastric distress at dosages greater than 40 mg/kg/day.

Decreased hearing that returns to normal after discontinuation of the drug has been reported several times. Alteration of normal flora is generally not a problem, but oral or perianal candidiasis occasionally develops. Transient cholestatic hepatitis is a rare complication that occurs with approximately equal frequency among the various formulations of erythromycin, but the estolate is said to pose a particular risk to pregnant women. Intramuscular administration of erythromycin is painful and irritative. IV doses should be administered slowly (1–2 hr).

Clindamycin and lincomycin can cause nausea, vomiting and diarrhea. Pseudomembranous colitis due to suppression of normal flora and overgrowth of *Clostridium difficile* is uncommon, especially in children, but potentially serious. Urticaria, glossitis, pruritis and skin rashes occur occasionally. Serum sickness, anaphylaxis and photosensitivity are rare as are hematologic and hepatic abnormalities.

The newer macrolides, azithromycin and clarithromycin, are less likely than erythromycin to cause gastrointestinal side effects.

Polymyxins. Polymyxin B and polymyxin E (colistin sulfate and colistimethate) are mainly of historic interest and are rarely used now except in topical preparations. With parenteral administration the major toxicity is to the kidneys. They also cause various neurological reactions such as flushing, dizziness, ataxia, diplopia, dysphagia, and paresthesias. Neuromuscular blockade with respiratory arrest has occurred. Hematologic or hepatic toxicity has rarely been attributed to the polymyxins. Oral colistin sulfate is well tolerated with few side effects.

Antituberculous Drugs. Isoniazid is generally well tolerated and hypersensitivity reactions are rare. Peripheral neuritis (preventable or reversed by pyridoxine administration) and mental aberrations from euphoria to psychosis occur more often in adults than in children. Mild elevations of ALT in the first weeks of therapy, which disappear with continued administration, are common. Rarely, frank hepatitis develops. Rifampin also can cause hepatitis; it is more common in patients with pre-existing liver disease or in those taking large dosages. Risk of hepatic damage increases when rifampin and isoniazid are taken together in dosages more than 15 mg/kg of each daily. Gastrointestinal, hematologic and neurologic side effects of various types have been observed on occasion. Hypersensitivity reactions are rare. Pyrazinamide can cause hepatic damage, which appears to be dose-related. Ethambutol has the potential for ocular damage.

Antifungal Drugs. Amphotericin B, flucytosine, miconazole, ketoconazole and itraconazole can produce serious adverse reactions. Amphotericin B is probably the most toxic antimicrobial drug in clinical use. Chills, fever, flushing and headaches are the most common of the many adverse reactions. Some degree of decreased renal function occurs in up to 80% of patients given amphotericin B. Anemia is common and, rarely, hepatic toxicity and neutropenia occur. Patients should be monitored for hypokalemia and hyponatremia.

The major toxicity of flucytosine is bone marrow depression, which is dosage-related, especially in patients treated concomitantly with amphotericin B. It also occurs in patients with a pre-existing hematologic disorder and in those treated with irradiation or cancer chemotherapeutic drugs. Mild gastrointestinal upset, mental confusion and vertigo sometimes occur. Renal function should be monitored.

There has been little experience with the parenteral preparation of miconazole in children but it appears to be only slightly less toxic than amphotericin B. Patients receiving miconazole should be monitored for hematologic, hepatic and renal toxicity.

Ketoconazole has produced hepatic damage on rare occasions. The most common side effect is gastric distress; this can often be alleviated by dividing the daily dose. Gynecomastia is not rare in adult males. Itraconazole has a smaller incidence of adverse effects than ketoconazole.

Fluconazole is usually well tolerated. Gastrointestinal symptoms, rash and headache occur occasionally. Transient, asymptomatic elevations of hepatic enzymes have been reported.

Vancomycin. Vancomycin can cause phlebitis if the drug is injected rapidly or in concentrated form. Vancomycin is said to have the potential for ototoxicity and nephrotoxicity, but documenting these effects in children is difficult. It was reported that vancomycin potentiated the nephrotoxicity of aminoglycosides but further study showed that this was probably incorrect. Hepatic toxicity is rare. Neutropenia has been reported. If the drug is infused too rapidly, a transient rash of the upper body with itching may occur from histamine release ("red man syndrome"). It is not a contraindication to continued use and is less likely if the infusion rate is 60–120 minutes. Vancomycin in conjunction with anesthesia has been reported to cause hypotension and hypothermia.

Sulfonamides and Trimethoprim. The most common adverse reaction to sulfonamides is a hypersensitivity rash. Rarely, Stevens-Johnson syndrome occurs; it was most common with very long-acting sulfas that are no longer marketed. The frequency and types of reactions to the trimethoprim-sulfamethoxazole combination are said to be the same as with sulfamethoxazole alone, but it is not clear whether Stevens-Johnson syndrome is caused more often by the combination than by sulfamethoxazole alone. Neutropenia and anemia occur occasionally. The rash caused by TMP/SMX appears to be more frequent in patients taking large dosages. Rash is common in adults with AIDS. Mild depression of platelet counts occurs in approximately one-half the patients treated with sulfas or trimethoprim-sulfamethoxazole but this rarely produces clinical bleeding problems. Sulfa drugs can precipitate hemolysis in patients with glucose-6-phosphate dehydrogenase deficiency. Crystalline aggregates of sulfa drugs may be deposited in the kidneys or ureters and cause acute nephropathy (most likely with sulfadiazine). Adequate urine output and alkalinization of the urine minimize the risk. Drug fever and serum sickness are infrequent hypersensitivity reactions. Hepatitis with focal or diffuse necrosis is rare. A rare idiosyncratic reaction to sulfa drugs is acute aseptic meningitis.

Fluoroquinolones. All quinolone and fluoroquinolone drugs cause cartilage damage in toxicity studies in various immature animals; however, no conclusive data indicate similar toxicity in young children. Studies to evaluate this have, to date, not found cartilage toxicity in children. Reported side effects include gastrointestinal symptoms, dizziness, headaches, tremors, confusion, seizures and rash. Hepatic toxicity is rare. Large dosages may precipitate hypoglycemia in the elderly. Severe hemolytic anemia occurred with temofloxacin with a frequency of approximately 1:10,000 patients; because of this the drug was withdrawn from the market.

Antiviral Drugs. After extensive clinical use, acyclovir has proved to be a safe drug with rare serious adverse effects. Renal dysfunction has occurred mainly with too rapid infusion of the drug. Rash, headache and gastrointestinal side effects are uncommon. There has been no controlled experience with the related drugs, famciclovir and valacyclovir, in children.

Amantadine produces dizziness, drowsiness and insomnia in many patients, but these effects are usually not severe. Visual disturbances, confusion, and psychosis are rare.

Foscarnet can cause renal dysfunction, anemia and cardiac rhythm disturbances. Seizures and neuropathy are other serious but rare toxicities. Ganciclovir causes hematologic toxicity. Gastrointestinal disturbances and neurologic damage are rarely encountered.

Vidarabine has been mainly replaced by acyclovir. A limiting factor to its use was the large volume of fluid required for its IV-administration which sometimes lead to fluid overload syndrome. It also causes nausea and vomiting, month and esophageal ulcerations and neurologic deficitis.

The many antiviral drugs for treatment for HIV infection have many adverse effects; consult the package inserts.

XVII. ADVERSE INTERACTIONS OF DRUGS

Antibiotic	Interacting Drug	Adverse Effect
Acyclovir	Probenecid	Poss incr acyclovir toxicity
Amantadine	Anticholinergics	Hallucinations, nightmares, confusion
Amikacin	(See Aminoglycosides)	
Aminoglycosides	Amphotericin B	Incr nephrotoxicity
	Anti-*Pseudomonas* penicillins (if renal failure)	Decr aminoglycoside serum conc
	Cephalosporins	Poss incr nephrotoxicity
	Digoxin	Poss decr digoxin effect
	Ethacrynic acid, furosemide, bumetanide	Incr ototoxicity
	Methotrexate	Poss incr methotrexate toxicity
	Neuromuscular blocking agents; magnesium sulfate	Incr neuromuscular blockage
Amphotericin B	Aminoglycosides	Incr nephrotoxicity
	Curariform drugs	Incr curariform effect
	Cyclosporine	Incr cyclosporine effect
	Digitalis drugs	Incr digitalis toxicity
	Miconazole	Decr anti-*Candida* effect
	Neuromuscular blocking agents	Hypokalemia
Ampicillin	Oral contraceptives	Decr contraceptive effect
	Allopurinol	Incr incidence of rash
Cephalosporins	Alcohol (cefamandole, cefoperazone, moxalactam)	Antabuse-like effect
	Aminoglycosides	Poss incr nephrotoxicity

Antibiotic	Interacting Drug	Adverse Effect
	Ethacrynic acid, furosemide	Incr nephrotoxicity
	Aspirin, heparin (moxalactam)	Poss incr bleeding risk
	Anticoagulants (moxalactam)	Incr anticoagulant effect
Chloramphenicol	Acetaminophen	Incr chloramphenicol toxicity
	Barbiturates	Incr barbiturate effect; Decr chloramphenicol effect
	Dicumarol	Incr anticoagulant effect
	Phenytoin	Altered pharmacology of both drugs
	Rifampin	Decr chloramphenicol effect
Ciprofloxacin	Theophylline, cyclosporine	Incr theophylline, cyclosporine
	Antacids	Decr ciprofloxacin absorption
Clindamycin, Lincomycin	Neuromuscular blocking agents	Incr neuromuscular blockade
	Diphenoxylate-atropine	Incr diarrhea, colitis
Cycloserine	(See Isoniazid)	
Erythromycin	Anticoagulants	Incr anticoagulant effect
	Digoxin	Incr digoxin effect
	Theophylline	Incr theophylline effect
	Carbamazepine	Incr carbamazepine effect
	Seldane	Cardiotoxic
Furazolidone	Alcohol	Antabuse-like effect
	Alpha-adrenergic amines	Incr hypertensive effect

Antibiotic	Interacting Drug	Adverse Effect
Gentamicin	(See Aminoglycosides)	
Griseofulvin	Oral anticoagulants	Decr anticoagulant effect
	Phenobarbital	Decr griseofulvin effect
Isoniazid	Aluminum antacids	Decr isoniazid effect
	Anticoagulants	Poss incr anticoagulant effect
	Carbamazepine	Incr toxicity of both drugs
	Cycloserine	Dizziness, drowsiness
	Phenytoin	Incr phenytoin toxicity
	Rifampin	Incr hepatotoxicity
Kanamycin	(See Aminoglycosides)	
Ketoconazole	Antacids	Decr ketoconazole effect
	Cimetidine	Decr ketoconazole effect
	Cyclosporine	Incr cyclosporine effect
	Erythromycin	Cardiotoxic
Lincomycin	(See Clindamycin)	
Metronidazole	Alcohol	Antabuse-like reaction
	Anticoagulants	Incr anticoagulant effect
	Phenobarbital	Decr metronidazole effect
Miconazole	(See Amphotericin B)	
Nalidixic acid	Oral anticoagulants	Incr anticoagulant effect
Netilmicin	(See Aminoglycosides)	
Quinacrine	Alcohol	Antabuse-like effect

Antibiotic	Interacting Drug	Adverse Effect
Rifampin	Anticoagulants, barbiturates, beta-adrenergic blockers, contraceptives, corticosteroids, diazepam, digitoxin, hypoglycemics, quinidine	Decreased effect of interacting drug
	Chloramphenicol	Decr chloramphenicol effect
	Isoniazid	Incr hepatotoxicity
	Methadone	Methadone withdrawal symptoms
Spectinomycin	Lithium	Incr lithium toxicity
Streptomycin	(See Aminoglycosides)	
Sulfonamides	Oral anticoagulants	Incr anticoagulant effect
	Hypoglycemics	Incr hypoglycemia
	Methotrexate	Poss incr methotrexate toxicity
	Phenytoin	Incr phenytoin effect
	Thiopental	Incr thiopental effect
Tetracyclines	Antacids, bismuth subsalicylate, iron, zinc sulfate	Decr tetracycline effect
	Phenytoin, barbiturates and carbamazepine	Decr doxycycline effect
	Oral contraceptives	Decr contraceptive effect
	Lithium	Incr lithium toxicity
Thiabendazole	Theophylline	Incr theophylline effect
Tobramycin	(See Aminoglycosides)	
Trimethoprim-sulfamethoxazole	Anticoagulants	Incr anticoagulant effect
Troleandomycin	Carbamazepine	Incr carbamazepine effect
	Oral contraceptives	Jaundice
	Theophylline	Incr theophylline effect
Vidarabine	Allopurinol	Incr vidarabine toxicity

XVIII. INDEX OF DISEASES

- D-

- E -

- F-

- G-